"Amy's wonderful writing style and humor make this a very enjoyable read. She shares her knowledge, research and personal journey in a way that empathizes with our challenges. I found many of Amy's tips and strategies to be insightful and helpful. The Stall Slayer is a must read."

—WENDY M.

"This book was very enlightening! After losing 25 pounds, I stalled in my weight loss for 6 weeks. After reading Amy's book, I am now losing weight again. Kudos for providing a realistic view that the process of adopting a low carb/high fat lifestyle takes educating ourselves to the research available plus plenty of support from those who are ahead of us in this journey!"

—CHERYL H.

"In a word? Excellent! It's one of the best resources I've read on this subject since my journey began in October 2018. This book is chock-full with practical, effective information. It's a goldmine of tips and suggestions backed by experience and sound science. In addition, the author's prose engages the reader and creates a comfortable environment for learning more about a sometimes frustrating topic. I felt like she was speaking directly to me rather than the often-clinical, structured, and lecture-type prose presented in some other books. It was a pleasure to read. Without a doubt, I know that many low-carbers will find hope, understanding, and answers to common challenges. I feel that all of the topics were relevant and important; nothing was 'filler.' Every section was bang-on and just made sense. Without question, this book will remain a trusted reference for me and a recommended resource for family and friends who encounter obstacles in their low-carb journey."

—JACOB L.

"I have a new understanding of thyroid hormones and function and how to interpret my thyroid panel results. This alone was worth more than the price of this book. Another highlight of this book is the chapter on an 'Information Vacation.' This is a wonderful idea. Time to shut out the noise for a little while. Finding a couple of authors, doctors and speakers as my role models and sticking to those like-minded individuals for a little while I think will be beneficial."

—JENNIFER B.

"The book was easy to read. I have been doing keto for a year and a half and quickly realized I was battling 'carb creep' and eating too much fat. Thanks for getting me back on track. I am tracking the carbs and was really surprised at how quickly they added up. Definitely carb creep. Thanks for writing the book and including that very important chapter. I expect to see changes!"

—NANCY R.

The Stall Slayer

Seven Roadblocks to Keto Fat Loss and What to Do About Them

Amy Berger, MS, CNS

Gutsy Badger Publishing
CHEYENNE, WYOMING

Amy Berger
Email: tuitnutrition@gmail.com
Visit www.tuitnutrition.com

The Stall Slayer / Amy Berger

ISBN 978-1-943721-15-3 (Paperback)
ISBN 978-1-943721-16-0 (Electronic)

Table of Contents

Disclaimer

Amy Berger, MS, CNS, is not a physician and Tuit Nutrition, LLC is not a medical practice. The information in this book is not intended as medical advice. It is not intended to diagnose, treat, cure, or prevent any disease or medical condition. It is not a substitute for care and treatment by a licensed medical professional.

Readers of this book hereby release Amy Berger, MS, CNS and Tuit Nutrition, LLC from any and all liability regarding the outcome to their health and/or weight upon implementation of any of the dietary and/or lifestyle suggestions contained herein. The information contained herein pertains to diet and lifestyle. It is not medical treatment and is not intended as such. Readers of this book are hereby instructed and encouraged to consult with their physicians and other licensed healthcare providers before embarking on any changes to their diet, lifestyle, nutritional supplementation and/or medication.

Links to websites, videos, graphics, scientific literature, and all other links are current as of the time of publication of this book. Inclusion of such links are for informational purposes only and are not to be considered endorsements of any other content on the site/domain, or by the author(s) and content creator(s) in question.

Introduction

As a keto-friendly nutritionist, stalled fat loss is one of the most common reasons people contact me for help. Every week I get multiple inquiries from people who've started a ketogenic diet and have either not lost any weight at all, or who lost a bit at first but whose weight hasn't budged in weeks or months. This can be demoralizing and disheartening when the internet is full of astonishing before and after photos and it 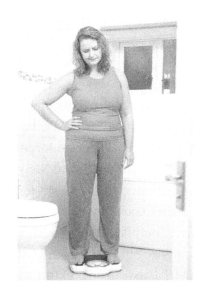 seems like weight is magically melting off everyone but you.

It's maddening when you think you're doing everything right and the scale isn't moving. You spend every free second lurking on forums and scrolling through Instagram feeds where people post miraculous-seeming weight loss transformations, trying to figure out what they're doing that you're not.

What are their macros? Do they fast? What about exercise? Do they take any supplements? What about MCT oil or exogenous ketones? Do they eat fat bombs? Drink fatty coffees? When you see someone getting the results you're working so hard for and *not* getting, it's only natural to want to know all their secrets. If you do exactly what they're doing, it'll work for you, too, right? It *has to*.

Not so fast.

As human beings, we all have a lot more in common than we have different. Much more unites us than divides us, especially when we're talking about the biochemistry and physiology of the human body. Black, White, Asian, African, Hispanic, Christian, Muslim, Jewish, Hindu, Buddhist, tall, short, male, female, blonde, brunette, or redhead: we all have kidneys, we all have a liver, we all have a pancreas. We all make cholesterol. And we can all burn fat and make ketones.

But that doesn't mean we're exactly the same. We have different genetics, different medical and dietary histories, hormone levels, stress loads, geographic environments, and other factors that affect metabolism and weight regulation. This means that just because something works for someone else doesn't mean it's going to work equally well for you. Learning from other people's success is a good place to start and can be helpful, but ultimately, you have to figure out what's going to work for *you*.

If I had to make an estimate, I'd say about 80% of the time I spend with clients is devoted to mythbusting and setting the record straight about how keto works. Low carb and ketogenic diets have exploded in popularity the last few years, which is great to see. And because they're so popular, there's a ton of information out there about them now—much more than there was when I was new to this. Unfortunately, along with all the good and trustworthy information, there's a lot of misleading nonsense and *mis*information that can lead people astray. If you're new to this, it can be hard to know what's reliable and what's better off ignored.

With that in mind, before I go any further, I should probably tell you a little about myself and how I got into all this.

My Story

I've been following a carb-restricted way of eating for over fifteen years. I'm not always strictly ketogenic, but I'm always low carb.

I bounce in and out of ketosis naturally, depending on what I'm eating or *not* eating, but I don't always aim to be in a state of deep ketosis by keeping carbs extremely low. I guess the best way to say it is, I never have a breakfast of pancakes and orange juice, but I'm not afraid of carrots and I don't think a tablespoon of hummus once in a while is going to kill me. I'm always fat-adapted—that is, my carbs are always low enough that I'm not riding the blood sugar and insulin rollercoasters anymore, and I can go several hours comfortably without eating, and I don't get irritable, shaky, or "hangry"—the combination of hungry and angry most of us remember very well from our life before keto. So I'm always low carb; sometimes ketogenic, sometimes not.

I started eating low carb primarily for fat loss. I was a chubby kid who grew into an overweight teenager and then into an overweight young adult. I was a couch potato as a child—my favorite activity was to curl up on a comfy couch with a book and read. (It still is.) Plus, my parents—*get this*—owned an ice cream store. I was literally "a kid in a candy store." Put those two together and you have a blueprint for a chubby child.

As I got older, I became unhappy with my size and shape. (Show me a girl raised in the 1980s and 1990s who *wasn't*.) In an attempt to lose weight, I became more physically active and paid attention to my diet. I even took up running (okay, to be honest, it was really more of a slow jog), and doubled-down on cutting fat out of my diet.

I did what I thought were "all the right things"—I did lots of exercise and ate my share of whole grains (whole wheat toast with light margarine was a frequent breakfast, as was fat-free cereal with skim milk), brown rice, low-fat or fat-free yogurt, pasta, and I knew I was doing good for myself by *baking* frozen breaded chicken nuggets & fries instead of frying them in oil. (Ha! If I knew then what I know now...) I snacked on cereal, pretzels, granola bars, crackers, and other low- and no-fat foods.

Despite the increased exercise, I didn't lose weight. In fact, very, *very* much increased exercise didn't do it for me either. At one point in my early twenties, I was unemployed and had lots of free time on my hands. I exercised twice a day, two hours in the morning and another two hours at night, and I *still* had no fat loss. I even trained for and completed a marathon, thinking there was *no way* I could do all that running and not lose weight. Well, the joke was on me, and I have the pudgy finish line photos to prove it! (In fact, I didn't learn the lesson well enough the first time and I ran a *second* marathon before it sunk in that running wasn't the answer to making me magically thin.)

I was fortunate that the only thing driving me toward low carb was weight loss. I had no health issues that I knew of at the time, but I have a family history of obesity, type 2 diabetes (T2D), cancer, and stroke, so the deck was stacked against me. There's no doubt in my mind that if I hadn't found low carb when I did, and if I'd kept on eating the way I had when I was younger—even though I *thought* I had a healthy diet—now I would likely be living with T2D, PCOS, obesity, and who knows what else.

I stumbled into the world of low carb via the book, *Dr. Atkins' New Diet Revolution.* (This was an updated version

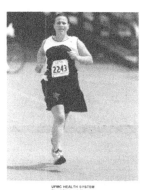

Me, running the Pittsburgh Marathon, 2001. Thanks for nothing, carb loading!

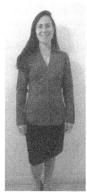

Me, 2014. Still exercising regularly, but diet was the biggest change - a *low carb* diet.

of *Dr. Atkins' Diet Revolution*, a.k.a. "the Atkins book," originally published in 1972.) My mother had picked it up at a yard sale! (Do people even still have those?) She never got around to reading it, but I did.

The Atkins book *made sense*. It was different—*very different*—from everything I thought I knew about nutrition and especially about how to lose weight. But since everything "I knew" had gotten me exactly nowhere, I figured I had nothing to lose by giving it a try—except a few pounds, maybe! You know what they say: "It's so crazy, it just might work."

This was around 1999, still smack-dab in the middle of the low-fat era, when "everyone knew" red meat, butter, egg yolks, and bacon were a heart attack waiting to happen. I remember the first time I put heavy cream in my coffee instead of skim milk: it was so rich and luxurious; I remember wondering if I would be able to feel it clogging my arteries immediately or if it would take a little while before it killed me. Well, 20 years later, here I am with no indicators whatsoever that my cardiovascular system is about to give out. (In case you're wondering why the math doesn't add up here, I didn't actually *stick with* low carb for the long term until 2003. I was in college in 1999 and I guess I just wasn't prepared to make that kind of change permanently. It took a few more

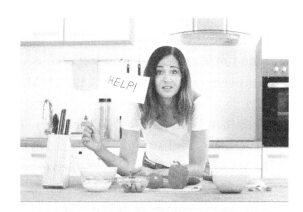

Confused and overwhelmed? I don't blame you!

7

years for it to sink in that my body simply doesn't do well with lots of starch and sugar—and that no amount of running would overcome that.)

When I first started learning about low carb, there was only *one* online forum and two or three books—that I knew of, anyway. A couple of books about diets high in fat and protein were published in the 1960s and even earlier (as far back as the 1800s, actually), but none ever attained the popularity of the Atkins book. (The other books I knew of at the time were *Protein Power*—still an excellent read, and *The Schwarzbein Principle.*)

The fact that there was so much less information about low carb and keto back then can be seen as a blessing and a curse. There was less information, but there was also less of that misleading and potentially counterproductive *misinformation*. Sometimes less is more, and that was certainly the case here. I don't envy you if you're new to this right now. The sheer amount of information—the websites, blogs, videos, forums, and feeds—can be totally overwhelming, especially because a lot of it contradicts itself. You read something on one person's blog, and someone else says the complete opposite in a video the next day. I'm not sure I would be able to sort through it all and even *get started* if I were brand new now. So, if you feel confused, stressed out, frustrated, and overwhelmed, you're not alone! (More on this issue in chapter 12.)

When I was new to this, there were no blood or breath ketone meters. MCT oil was not available to the general public. You had to be in a scientific study if you wanted to get supplemental exogenous ketones, and you couldn't drink them; researchers had to infuse beta-hydroxybutyrate directly into your blood. Coconut oil wasn't sold at most supermarkets in the US because there was basically no market for it back then—who in their right mind would buy a jar of mostly saturated fat? (Are you *trying* to kill yourself?!) There were no "macro calculators," no fat bomb recipes, and Facebook, Instagram, Twitter, and Reddit *didn't even exist.*

I didn't understand as much of the biochemistry and physiology around keto as I do now, but the thing is, you don't *have to* understand the science for keto to work for you. All I knew was that I needed to keep my carbs really low. I didn't need to count calories, weigh or measure my food, or do much of *anything* besides keeping my total carbohydrate intake very low. I followed the Atkins plan as originally written, *and it worked.* I used the urine test strips to make sure my carbs were low enough to keep me in ketosis, and what do you know...*fat loss!* No more obsessively thinking about my next meal. No more sugar cravings. No more fantasizing about food all day. I was born and raised in New York City and I haven't had a bagel in over a decade.

My point is, long before I studied nutrition formally and became a professional nutritionist, I had success with low carb. Long before I had a deeper understanding of the metabolic processes and biochemical feedback loops responsible for oxidizing fat and glucose, or storing and mobilizing fat, I did *just fine.* You need to understand only

> The sheer amount of information—the websites, blogs, videos, forums, and feeds—can be totally overwhelming, especially because a lot of it contradicts itself. You read something on one person's blog, and someone else says the complete opposite in a video the next day. If you feel confused, stressed out, frustrated, and overwhelmed, you're not alone!

a few fundamental principles in order for this way of eating to work for you. You don't need a PhD and you don't need to go to medical school. You don't need apps, meters, food scales, or any other high-tech gadgets, although these things do have their place in certain circumstances, and I'll cover those later on. Overall, though, as with so many things in life, the truth is, the most effective approach is to keep it simple.

In the chapters that follow, I'll walk you through the most common roadblocks to fat loss on ketogenic or low carb diets, and *what to do about them*. I'll provide some basic information on how and why ketogenic diets work when your goal is fat loss, dispel some myths that might be interfering with your fat loss goals, and offer advice on how to course-correct to start getting the results you want. Sometimes all it takes is a small change for things to start going more smoothly.

1
Is It Really a Stall?

When you're trying to break a fat loss stall, the first step is to figure out whether you're *actually stalled*. If it's only been a few days or weeks since you've lost any weight, I have news for you: you're not stalled. Stalls or plateaus in fat loss are not measured in days or even weeks, but in *months*.

It's important to understand that fat loss is not linear. You don't lose a little bit every day, steadily, until you magically arrive at your goal weight. *If only, right?!* There will be bumps and hiccups along the way—slight ups and downs, and days and weeks where the scale doesn't change at all. This is *completely normal*, and you have to be mentally prepared for it. Going a few days or even a few weeks without any change on the scale is not a stall; it's your complicated and complex human body being complicated and complex.

Over the course of the months, years, or decades that you *gained* weight to get to where you are now, it's unlikely that you gained a couple of ounces steadily every single day until reaching your highest weight. It's more likely that it came on a bit at a

> Fat loss is not linear. You don't lose a little bit every day, steadily, until you magically arrive at your goal weight. There will be bumps and hiccups along the way—slight ups and downs, and days and weeks where the scale doesn't change at all. This is *completely normal.*

time, stayed steady for a while, then increased a little more, stayed the same for another while, increased a bit more, and so on. The reason you didn't *see* it going up a little bit once in a while and then staying the same for weeks or months is because *you weren't getting on the scale every day.* So, just like you didn't *gain* a little weight every single day in a steady pattern, most of us don't *lose* weight every single day in a steady pattern. There'll be a bit of loss, then some amount of time at a steady weight, then a little bit of loss again, then another period of time at a steady weight, maybe a little bit of weight *gain*, then some loss again...

Wait a minute. Weight *gain?* Did she just say weight *gain?*

Yes. Yes, I did.

Before you freak out, stay with me.

HOW YOU *WANT* WEIGHT LOSS TO WORK

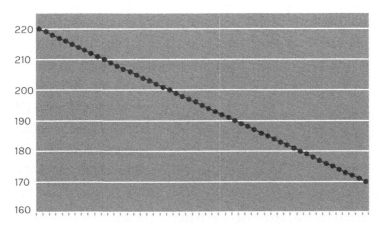

TIME (WEEKS, MONTHS, YEARS)

HOW WEIGHT LOSS *REALLY* WORKS

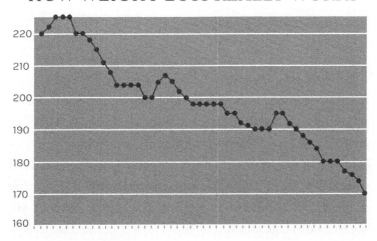

TIME (WEEKS, MONTHS, YEARS)

Not By Scale Alone

Don't go solely by the scale when assessing how keto is working for you. The scale is only one tool among many that can give you information about how your body is changing from this way of eating, and it's probably the most misleading. Keep in mind that scales measure only body weight, and you don't want to lose *weight*, you want to lose *fat*. When you're using keto (or any other eating plan) for the purpose of losing body fat, it's not uncommon for your *size and shape* to change even when your *scale weight* stays the same—or even goes *up a little!* When this happens, your clothing will fit differently. Your waist might be shrinking. If you wear rings, they might be looser. For this reason—changes in body size and shape even when the scale doesn't budge—a tape measure and your clothing are often better tools than a scale for assessing changes to your body.

> Don't go solely by the scale when assessing how keto is working for you. The scale is only one tool among many that can give you information about how your body is changing from this way of eating, and it's the most misleading.

Take your measurements once a week or twice a month. Not just your belly, waist, and hips, but also your upper arms, thighs, calves, neck, or anywhere else you'd like, particularly if you're looking to lose a large amount of fat. (This applies less to those who are already close to their goal weight or shape. These changes will be less noticeable for those people.) Notice how your clothes are fitting. **If your measurements are changing, *you are not stalled.***

I recommend weighing yourself no more often than once a week, and once every *two* weeks would be even better—if you choose to weigh yourself at all. Some people prefer to weigh themselves daily, and I understand that. They find that it helps keep them accountable and stay on top of things: if they weigh themselves every day, they can catch weight gain in the early stage, before it creeps up very high. It's easier to course-correct and get back on track when it's just a little snowball of a couple pounds coming back on as opposed to an all-out avalanche of regaining everything you'd lost and then some.

I don't recommend weighing yourself every day, so if you're not doing that, don't start. If you *are* a chronic weigher, though, and you want to *keep* weighing daily, there are some things you need to understand and have at the front of your mind every time you step on the scale. (These apply to people who weigh themselves only once in a while, too.)

- **Weight versus fat:** Scales measure only *weight*, not *fat*. A regular ol' bathroom scale does not know the difference between water, muscle mass, organs, tendons, ligaments, bones, and body fat. It cannot distinguish between any of these. Scales measure one thing and one thing only: the force of Earth's gravity on your physical body. (That's what your weight is, in the technical sense.) A bioimpedance scale can measure body fat, water weight, and other tissue mass, but if you're using one that was relatively inexpensive and looks like most regular bathroom scales, I wouldn't take the results as gospel. Some doctors' offices and gyms have more reliable (and more expensive) models that will give you more accurate results if you insist on tracking things to this degree. Bottom line: *Your body weight doesn't tell you how much body fat you're carrying.*

- **Water weight:** Scale weight can fluctuate by as much as 2-3 pounds from day to day, and this does not necessarily reflect a change in body *fat*. The short list of things that affect weight in the short term—and remember, this is just the short list—includes environmental humidity, sodium intake, exercise, and hormonal changes, particularly for women during the menstrual cycle. (Gotta love those hormones, right ladies?) Not everyone retains water when they consume a lot of sodium (salt), but some people do, and this can affect scale weight. Most people retain a bit of water when it's humid out, and, surprisingly, when they exercise. Exercise can be helpful for building muscle mass and maintaining fat loss, but in the short term, physical exertion—especially weightlifting or resistance training—can make the muscles hang onto water, causing your scale weight to stay the same or possibly even go *up* a little. I hope it's obvious that this not because you gained body fat. It's just water, and it won't stay around long. I understand it can be frustrating as all you-know-what when you don't see your scale weight decrease, or maybe it even *increases*, but this is why I recommend against weighing every day. An increase in the number on the scale because of water weight does not mean you have gained body fat. *Water retention is not a fat loss stall.*

- **Gaining good weight:** This might apply more to women than men, but it'll apply to some dudes out there, too. If you've spent several years (maybe close to your whole life!) restricting calories, over-exercising, undereating, and living on low- and no-fat foods that were high in carbohydrate (things we all *thought* were "good for us" – granola bars, bran muffins, fat-free yogurt, soy lattes), your body likely lost some very important tissue it couldn't afford to hold onto when you were pushing yourself to the limits without adequate rest and nutritional replenishment. Now that you're feeding yourself better foods—good quality proteins and fats—and your body is actually *being nourished*, you might be rebuilding critical tissue you lost during all the years your body wasn't getting what it needed. You could be replacing lost bone mass and muscle mass, or strengthening connective tissue

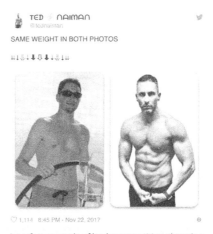

TED NAIMAN
@tednaiman

SAME WEIGHT IN BOTH PHOTOS

♡ 1,114 8:45 PM · Nov 22, 2017

A perfect example of body composition changing dramatically while scale weight stays the same. This is Ted Naiman, MD, a keto-friendly doctor in the Seattle area. (Image used with permission.)

such as tendons and ligaments. This is a *good thing*, but it might show itself in either no downward movement on the scale, or possibly even a little *increase* in your weight. Just because the scale isn't moving, or isn't moving as quickly as you'd like it to, doesn't mean good things aren't happening inside you—things that *need* to happen if you want to age gracefully and be able to get up out of a chair under your own power when you're 85, or to not break a hip if you take a fall when you're 70. Let me say that again for the folks in the back: *just because your scale weight isn't changing doesn't mean very good, very important things aren't happening inside you.* **Weight gain due to building muscle or bone mass is not a fat loss stall.**

- **Menstrual cycle:** Ladies, you have *got* to stop driving yourselves crazy over fluctuations of only a couple pounds from day to day when you're of reproductive age and are riding the hormone rollercoaster. Many women report that keto helps tremendously with PMS symptoms, and that their mood swings, irritability, cravings, breast tenderness, cramps, skin breakouts, and other issues are massively improved since going keto. But this isn't true for everyone, and a little bit of bloating around "that time" is totally normal, keto or not. I can't stress this enough: remember that it's just water and it'll be gone as soon as Aunt Flo leaves. *Premenstrual bloating and water retention are not a fat loss stall.*

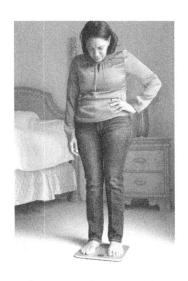

Pre-menstrual water retention is not a stall.

Another tip—well, more like a personal plea—for those who insist on weighing themselves every day: don't use the scale as the judge of whether you are a good, lovable, worthy human being. Those qualities have nothing—*nothing*—to do with your size, shape, or weight. (They also have nothing to do with how "keto" you are, how many carbs you're eating, or how "clean" your diet is.) Do not let the number you see on that blasted scale determine whether you have a good or bad day, what kind of mood you'll be in, or whether you deserve to have a happy, fulfilling life. If the scale has this amount of power over you, *take that power back*. Take a sledgehammer to your scale and show it who's boss. (Or at the very least, stash it away out of sight, at the back of a very deep, dark closet, where it belongs, and *forget about it for a while*.)

What if it Really *is* a Stall?

If it's been 2 or 3 months—yes, *months*—and there's been no change in your weight *or* your measurements, *or* your body composition, *or* how your clothing fits, maybe it really is a stall. If so, now what?

> Even if your weight and measurements aren't changing, good things are happening *on the inside.*

If you *are* truly stalled, I have two bits of good news for you:

First: Know that even if your weight and measurements aren't changing, good things are happening on the inside. As long as your carbs are low, which keeps your blood sugar and insulin on the low side, you're reaping the cardiometabolic benefits of this way of eating. You can have lower triglycerides, higher HDL, lower inflammation, better energy levels, less acid reflux, less joint pain, clearer skin, fewer cravings, sharper thinking, more stable moods, and less insatiable hunger *even if you haven't lost any weight.* Researchers have shown that the cardiovascular and metabolic benefits of carbohydrate restriction occur even in the absence of fat loss.[1,2] This means that people get healthier on keto even when they don't lose weight.

This makes sense, right? Not everyone who adopts a ketogenic diet does it for the purpose of losing body fat, so we know keto does a lot of good for a lot of other reasons. People use this way of eating as a treatment for epilepsy, for lowering blood sugar and insulin in type 2 diabetes, for improving hormone levels and restoring fertility in polycystic ovarian syndrome (PCOS), reversing non-alcoholic fatty liver disease (NAFLD), for enhancing athletic performance, for blasting away brain fog, reducing frequency and severity of migraines, getting rid of acid reflux/

GERD, and there's exciting research emerging that keto can help people living with Parkinson's and Alzheimer's diseases. Keto is also very helpful for people with type 1 diabetes.[3-20] (These folks will always require at least some insulin from injections, but keto can dramatically reduce the doses they need, which helps reduce the likelihood of dangerous hypo- and hyperglycemia, and the long-term complications of type 1 diabetes.) The bottom line here is, people use keto for many different reasons besides fat loss, and not everyone who does keto is or was overweight or obese, so we know that keto can be great for the body even when weight loss isn't part of the picture.

> As long as your carbs are low, which keeps your blood sugar and insulin on the low side, you're reaping the cardiometabolic benefits of this way of eating even if you aren't losing weight.

Stay the course and trust the process. If you're eating keto, you're getting healthier on the inside, even if you don't see it on the outside just yet.

Second: The second bit of good news is that stalls are fixable! You're stalled, not stuck. Stalls are temporary, not permanent. Your fat loss isn't stopped; it's just on hold for a bit.

There's a great saying that will serve you well to keep in mind as you read the rest of this book: "What got you here won't get you there." You might have been lean, healthy, and energetic on a steady diet of pizza, fries, sugary sodas, bagels, and breakfast cereal when you were 17 or 27 years old. But maybe that stopped working so well when you were 47, or 57, or 67, and you found keto somewhere along the way. In the same sense, the version of keto you started with and that worked well at first might not be what you need *now*.

Maybe the amounts of carbs, fat, and protein that worked at the beginning need a little tweaking now. If you're a woman, maybe you're going through menopause or you're already done with it, and the hormonal changes are making it harder to lose weight than when you were younger. Maybe you've gotten a little too generous with keto treats or you're eating more carbs than you realize. Maybe your thyroid is a bit wonky and suboptimal hormone levels are standing in the way of fat loss even though you're as strict as ever with your diet and exercise.

If you've already come a long way in your fat loss, or maybe not all that long a way just yet, but you're genuinely stalled now, take heart. This book will help you figure out *why* your fat loss has paused and *how to get it moving again*.

2
Setting Your Expectations

Having read chapter 1, if you've determined that your fat loss is really, truly stalled, the next step is to determine whether you actually *should* be looking to lose body fat. Are you carrying excess body fat to the point that 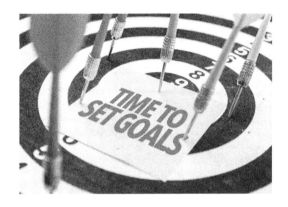 it's interfering with your health, mobility, and quality of life, or are you already close to your goal weight and looking to lose "the last few pounds?" Is it possible you're actually *already* at a perfectly suitable weight or body fat percentage for your age and sex, but you don't realize this? Trying to lose body fat when you're already "there" is an exercise in frustration and futility. To save you heartache and banging your head against the wall, let's talk about setting reasonable expectations.

Slow Fat Loss is *Still* Fat Loss

Fat loss is not a race. Losing body fat slowly is *still losing body fat*. Don't compare your results to anyone else's. This is easier said than done, I know. It's easy to look at other people's before & after photos and feel jealous, or be angry, disappointed, and frustrated that everyone is losing faster than you are.

Generally speaking, young people lose body fat faster than older folks, and men lose faster than women. People who've been overweight for only a short time tend to lose more easily than people who've been heavy most of their lives. These are generalizations, though. There are always exceptions.

Women, don't compare yourself to men. This is a one-way ticket to disappointment and resentment. (Like I said in chapter 1...gotta love those hormones!) Men typically lose weight more quickly and easily than women do, especially women in their peri- and post-menopausal years. We gals can and do lose body fat just fine on keto, but it often happens more slowly than it does for our husbands, brothers, fathers, sons, and male friends. (Lucky for them, we love them anyway.)

> Many people find keto to be faster and more effective for fat loss than any other approach they've ever tried, but that doesn't mean it's going to be as fast as you *want* it to be.

Women might also be dealing with other issues that can make fat loss more difficult—issues that affect men as well, but which are more common in women, such as hypothyroidism. (More on this in chapter 6.) And remember what I said in chapter 1—women are more likely than men to have histories of obsessive calorie restriction and under-consuming protein, and after adopting a ketogenic diet, they might be replacing some of that lost bone and muscle tissue. So when women see a small bump up on the scale, this isn't always body fat; it could be critically important *healthy weight* that you *want* to gain. Ladies, remember that your *shape* might be changing even if your scale weight stays the same or possibly even goes up a little. I know I sound like a broken record making this point over and over, but so many women are exclusively focused on the scale—to the point that it nearly runs (and ruins!) their life—and it's critically important that they understand the difference between *weight* and *fat*.

"Seasoned" and senior citizens, don't compare your rate of fat loss to people twenty, thirty, forty, or *fifty* years younger than you are. Even the healthiest people among us experience inevitable hormonal and metabolic changes as they get older, and these can make it more difficult to lose body fat. Not impossible, just more difficult than when they were younger.

Are Your Goals Realistic?

Doctors who use low carb and ketogenic diets in their clinics say that a reasonable rate of weight loss is about 1-2 pounds (0.5-1 kg) per week. But this depends on your starting weight, or, more precisely, your starting body fat percentage. The more you're looking to lose and the higher the amount of fat you carry, the more quickly it will come off—at first.

When you're new to keto, weight tends to come off quickly, especially if your starting weight is very high. It slows down after the first few days or weeks, but *this is normal.* You might have heard that the reason you lose so much weight on keto is because it's all "water weight." This is true, but only for the first few days. And just so we're clear here, losing water is great! You *want* to lose excess water your body is holding onto, especially if you have hypertension (high blood pressure), edema (fluid retention), or any other condition influenced by your body hanging onto too much water. The water comes off quickly, but it can take a bit more time for *fat* to leave the body.

Fat *will* leave, but you have to be patient. It won't leave as quickly as the water did. This slowdown in weight loss is to be expected, and you need to be mentally prepared for it, just like you have to be ready for the expected small blips up and down in scale weight. Play the long game. You didn't gain this fat overnight, and you're not going to lose it that quickly, either. Many people find keto to be faster and more effective for fat loss than any other approach they've ever tried, but that doesn't mean it's going to be as fast as you *want* it to be. Don't be discouraged by days or weeks where the scale doesn't move, or your clothes don't fit differently. Pay attention to the trends over time—the long-term changes and movement in the right direction, regardless of how small they are or how slowly they occur.

> Play the long game. You didn't gain this fat overnight, and you're not going to lose it that quickly, either.

The less fat you're looking to lose, the more difficult it often is to lose it. This means you might have to be stricter with your diet than someone who's looking to lose much more fat, and it might take more than just keto alone. We all know people who only had to "clean up" their diet a little in order to have seemingly effortless fat loss. (When I was in the Air Force, I knew guys who could stop drinking beer and lose ten pounds. No keto, no carb counting, no *nothing*. Just ditch beer and the weight fell off. *Sigh*.) Most of us aren't this lucky, and if you're already close to your goal weight or physique, it might take more effort to go those final steps.

Body Dysmorphia

The sad reality of life in the industrialized world in the 21st Century is that we have come to fetishize thinness. We are obsessed with being "lean," "ripped," "shredded," "cut," "toned," and whatever other words there are to describe the physiques many of us envy.

Scrolling through pictures on "fitspo" (fitness inspiration) accounts online or flipping through physique magazines can be motivating and inspiring for some people, but for others it's demoralizing, disheartening, and discouraging. We compare ourselves to people who might not even exist in real life. Not the way they look in those pictures, anyway. A fortune of money in professional lighting, makeup, photo editing, and maybe even cosmetic surgery go into erasing every last wrinkle, pore, line, age spot, scar, stretch mark, sag, bag, jiggle, and cellulite dimple. We will never measure up to doctored images that remove a model's humanness, and it's a waste of emotional energy to feel like we should.

With this in mind, do you have a realistic self-image? Do you see yourself the way others see you?

We often don't have an accurate sense of how we really look. For many of us, looking at ourselves in a mirror is like looking at a funhouse mirror—the ones that distort our size and shape to make us appear much shorter and wider or much taller and thinner than we actually are. Many of us have a wildly inaccurate sense of our own appearance and the size and shape of our bodies.

Thinking that you are much larger or much smaller than you actually are is called *body dysmorphia*. (This is different from body *dysphoria*, which is a sense of extreme unhappiness regarding your physical body. Body dysphoria can be a *result* of dysmorphia, but dysmorphia does not necessarily imply that you are unhappy with your physique. It means only that you do not have an accurate perception of your true shape and size.)

If you think you have body dysmorphia or you suspect that your self-perception regarding your body size might not be accurate, consider asking trusted friends or family members to give you their honest perspective. This can be a touchy subject, though. You need to have a thick skin for this. Be prepared for responses to run the gamut. Some you'll agree with; others might surprise you or possibly feel offensive or insulting to you. But if you're genuinely not sure whether you should even be trying to lose body fat at all, it might help to get input from people close to you, especially if they're familiar with your health, medical, and dietary histories, and if you trust them to be honest with you. Honest, but gentle. (Unless you *want* a tough love approach, in which case, tell them not to hold back. I don't recommend this unless you're tough as nails, though!) If you prefer, keep those relationships intact and work with a medical professional, nutritionist, or personal trainer to get a more precise measurement of your body fat percentage to help determine whether you're already at an appropriate level of body fat for your sex and age.

Sensible Ambition

It's good to be ambitious, but set a fat loss goal that is reasonable for you to attain. Remember that you're playing the long game. If you've been heavy for most of your life, it might not be wise to start out with a goal weight you've only fantasized about. Keep that ultimate destination in mind and let it drive you continually forward, but consider setting a smaller goal to start out with and once you get there, reassess and make a new goal. Think about how people climb Mount Everest: they don't start at the bottom and move up in altitude nonstop until they reach the summit. There are base camps located along the way where they stop to rest and acclimate for some period of time before moving on. If you have a substantial amount of weight to lose, think of each smaller goal along the way as a kind of base camp for yourself—a place for you to celebrate how far you've come and to make a game plan for what's next.

On the other hand, if you're looking to lose a relatively small amount of weight, this often tends to be more difficult than losing more. The closer you already are to your goal weight when you start out, the more your body sometimes fights to hang on to those last few pounds or body fat percentage points. This is where a phrase I once heard comes in. I wish I could remember who said it because I'd like to give them credit for it, but I don't remember where it came from, so thank you to the anonymous wise one: Keto can make you as lean as you can be, but that might not be as lean as you *want* to be.

What this means is, a nutritionally complete low carb or ketogenic diet with amounts of protein, fat, and carbohydrate that are appropriate for you can help you lose body fat and change your appearance to a great degree, but you might want to get even leaner or more "shredded" than keto alone can deliver. For example, if you want those elusive six-pack abs, even if you lose fat around your midsection, you won't have rippling muscles *if you don't have rippling muscles*. Losing fat and building muscle are not the same thing. Keto is great for the former. It can *help* with the latter, but the latter has a lot more to do with stressing your muscles so they have to strengthen and adapt to that stress than it does with not eating carbs.

> Keto can make you as lean as you can be, but that might not be as lean as you *want* to be.

Depending on what your ultimate goals are with regard to your size, shape, and physique, in order to have your dream body you might have to devote a lot more effort and go to extraordinary lengths beyond "just keto"—some of which might not be sustainable for the long-term. This is why it can be helpful to work with a professional to assess whether your goals are sensible, but even more importantly, whether they're *safe and healthy*.

An Uncomfortable Truth

Remember what I said about all that airbrushing and photo editing? Don't believe everything you see online. When we scroll through fitness and diet feeds online, we see only the highlight reels, not the outtakes. We see the six-pack abs, the toned triceps, the glowing smiles, the keto lasagna bursting with cheese... But the reality is, we don't know what goes on behind closed doors when the cameras are off and the phones are out of sight.

Things are not always what they seem. I hate to be the bearer of bad news, but you have a right to know the truth: there's a lot of disordered eating in the keto world, even among the professionals. (The same is true for Paleo, veganism, and just about any other dietary strategy that has a special name or set of rules.) You might *think* your favorite keto blogger, video maker, podcaster, or "personality" gets their results solely through grass-fed beef and organic broccoli, and from fair-trade coconut oil blended into their mold-free coffee, because they sure *look* amazing in all the pictures they post. Based on their smile, you'd think no human has ever been happier to see a pile of kale or a fried egg in their life.

But what you *don't* see is that the young woman you admire so much hasn't menstruated in a year, and the ripped guy whose Instagram feed you check every morning is anxious, depressed, and hasn't had an erection in 4 months. My point is, many people achieve their desired results through diet alone, but some don't. Some are going to extreme lengths to attain a certain physique— including employing ill-advised and even dangerous strategies to get there—and they're not being honest with you about it.

Whether it's in the form of severe long-term calorie restriction, exercise addiction, bingeing and purging (be this by vomiting, abusing laxatives, or "exercise bulimia"), or some other dangerous or disordered eating or exercise pattern, some of the people you follow in the keto world or in other diet communities may be going to great lengths to keep up an appearance they'd like you to believe is coming solely through their chosen diet. The result is that *you* end up feeling like a failure when the diet alone doesn't work equally well for you.

To be clear, diet alone does work for many people, so I'm not accusing everyone who looks like dynamite of being underhanded and dishonest. But this kind of problematic behavior does exist behind the scenes, and pretending it doesn't does all of us a disservice: it keeps the people enmeshed in it from getting the help they need, and it makes the rest of us feel like failures. We shouldn't envy people who have desirable physiques that came at the expense of their mental and emotional health.

What are You Willing to Do?

When setting your goals, ask yourself what you're willing to do. If you'd like to lose body fat, are you willing to keep carbs very low or possibly cut back a bit on dietary fat? If you want to get stronger or faster, are you willing to do the kind of training becoming stronger or faster requires? If you have a goal physique in mind, ask yourself if you're willing to do what it will take to get there, keeping in mind that keto alone might not be sufficient.

Check in with yourself periodically to assess whether you're satisfied with where you are in terms of your weight, size, and shape, or if you'd like to change in some way. This is especially important if you started out with a goal weight or body fat percentage—meaning, a precise number you

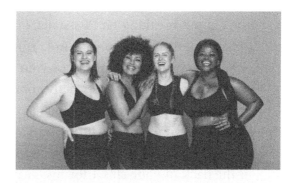

Maybe you're just fine exactly as you are *right now*.

were looking to get to. It's possible to get there and still be unhappy, or to *not* be there yet, but feel great and be perfectly content where you are. This is why it's important to assess things once in a while: you might surprise yourself, because *maybe you're already happy with things as they are, and you didn't even realize it.* You were waiting for a number on a scale or a body scan to tell you you'd "arrived" when you'd already been there for a while.

Because of these possibilities—reaching your goal weight and still being unhappy with your appearance, or being totally satisfied with your physique even if you're not at whatever goal number you set for yourself—I suggest not having a goal weight at all. Goals, yes. A goal *weight*, no. Remember what I said about body fat, water, muscle mass, bones, and all the other stuff that figures into scale weight: your *weight* doesn't tell you much about how you *look*, and certainly not a whole lot about how healthy you are.

> I suggest not having a goal weight at all. Goals, yes. A goal *weight*, no.

It's nearly impossible to recommend what kind of goal you should have. This is an entirely personal thing. You *can* have a goal weight in mind; I'm just trying to show you that this can be counterproductive. Since this is a book about breaking fat loss stalls, I'm not here to convince you to have a goal related to your mile run time, your triglyceride-to-HDL ratio, your bench press, or your hemoglobin A1c, although any of those might be a perfectly good thing to want to improve. You're reading this because you're concerned with fat loss. So, consider having a goal of fitting into a certain article of clothing—whether something brand new or something that's been hanging in the back of your closet for five years because that was the last time you could fit into it.

You don't have to have a goal other than fat loss. What I'm trying to impart to you is, if you do have a specific body fat percentage, weight, or physique goal in mind, consider working with a medical, fitness, or nutrition professional to determine whether it's safe, healthy, and sensible for you, and reassess from time to time to see if you should make any adjustments, or if things are actually just fine as they are.

3

The Macro Myth: How Keto *Really* Works

I have something shocking to tell you.

When you're using a ketogenic diet specifically for the purpose of losing body fat, there's no such thing as ketogenic ratios.

The ketogenic diet—very low in carbs, high in fat, and moderate in protein—was originally developed as a medical therapy for epilepsy. Specifically, it was developed in the 1920s, before there were anticonvulsant drugs and there were no effective treatments for this condition besides fasting. It was recognized as far back as ancient Greece that fasting seemed to reduce the frequency and severity of seizures in people with epilepsy. Ketogenic diets reproduce some of

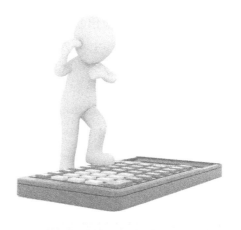

Your body is not a calculator.

the metabolic and physiologic changes that occur during fasting, and epilepsy is the condition for which there's currently the largest and most solid supporting body of scientific research for keto.[1-3] In fact, keto is still currently used by children and adults with epilepsy—especially those for whom most (or all!) of the anticonvulsant medications are ineffective.

However, using a ketogenic diet for fat loss is a totally different animal.

The ketogenic diet (KD) for epilepsy was originally designed with a 3:1 or 4:1 ratio of fat to protein and carbs *combined*. This means 3 or 4 grams of fat for every 1 gram of protein and/or carbohydrate—for every 5 grams of food consumed, there are 4 grams of fat and 1 gram of protein and/or carbs. This means that a 3:1 keto diet is 75% fat, while a 4:1 keto diet is 80% fat. It was initially believed that this very high amount of fat and a reduced protein intake was required for the diet to be effective. In the decades that have passed since the diet was originally developed, and based on results from thousands of patients, research indicates that not everyone requires this strict a diet and this degree of protein restriction. Some people with epilepsy experience wonderful seizure control on a modified Atkins diet (higher in protein), or even on diets that are slightly higher in carbs but where MCT oil makes up a larger proportion of the fat intake. Some people even do well without going keto at all, but just doing a gluten-free/casein-free diet.

Regardless of whatever variation of keto or low carb is effective for epilepsy, fat loss is a different ballgame. Implementing a nutritional strategy for fat loss is not the same as using a similar diet as therapy for a serious medical condition.

How Keto Works

Ketogenic diets are effective for improving a wide range of health issues because they induce a number of biochemical and hormonal changes in the body. I could fill an entire full-length book with the different mechanisms of keto and explain why those mechanisms make this way of eating effective for helping people with migraines, hypertension, gout, cardiovascular disease, types 1 and 2 diabetes, PCOS, Parkinson's disease, and more. But since I didn't want to make this a full-length book and you're reading it specifically because you want to break a fat loss stall, let's stick to why and how keto helps with losing body fat.

If you want to lose body fat, you have to *burn* body fat, and in order to burn body fat, you first have to get the fat out of where it's stored: in your fat cells (technically called *adipose* cells). It's like getting cash out of an ATM: pretend there are no such things as credit cards or buying things online. (I know, probably impossible to even imagine this, but stay with me here.) If you want to be able to pay for things with cash, first you have to go to an ATM and *get* some cash.

Getting fat out of your fat cells—making a withdrawal from your adipose ATM—should be easy. After all, that's what your stored fat is there for: to be used for energy when you don't have enough energy coming in from the outside. It's like your savings account: when you don't have enough cash flow coming in, you dip into your savings to tide you over until you do. The difference is, while you might not want to have to tap into your financial savings, your excess *fat* savings are stores you *do* want to dwindle down. (Note, though, that I said *excess* fat. We all need *some* body fat! Your body fat percentage should never be zero. In fact, you'd be dead long before you got there, and you'd feel pretty terrible, physically and mentally, as you got closer and closer. So you don't want to lose *all* your fat; just the amount that's either affecting your health, mobility, and quality of life, or enough to make you a little more pleased with what you see in the mirror.)

Getting back to the main message, getting fat out of your fat cells should be easy. Your body should release it when necessary. The problem for most of us is that it's *not* easy. Our bodies seem to want to hang on to every last ounce for dear life. It's as if there's an impenetrable forcefield surrounding our stored fat, keeping it locked exactly where it is.

In fact, this isn't too far off the mark, and it mostly has to do with the hormone insulin. You're probably used to thinking of insulin as a "blood sugar hormone," but insulin does so much more than that. It has a major influence on our ability to release and burn fat. Think of insulin as a security guard that stands outside your fat cells and makes sure no fat escapes. If you want to get stored fat out of those fat cells so it can be sent to other cells to be burned for fuel, you have to get insulin out of the way. And the way to do that is to limit intake of foods that raise insulin the most. For most people, this means refined carbohydrates, and for many, it means carbohydrates in general, even ones we might otherwise consider wholesome and nutritious, like sweet potatoes, beets, black beans, pineapple, and other starchy vegetables, beans, and fruit. It's not that these foods are "bad" for us, or that they're not nutritious. It's just that some of us are more sensitive to carbohydrate than others, even from these kinds of natural, whole foods.

Not everyone is carb-intolerant; after all, plenty of people eat lots of starch and sugar and aren't overweight and don't have health problems tied to insulin resistance or metabolic syndrome. But if you're following a ketogenic

> Think of insulin as a security guard that stands outside your fat cells and makes sure no fat escapes. If you want to get stored fat out of those fat cells so it can be sent to other cells as fuel to be burned, you have to get insulin out of the way. And the way to do that is to limit intake of foods that raise insulin the most.

diet to lose weight because other strategies you've tried haven't worked, such as a low-fat diet or increased exercise, then you're probably not one of those lucky carb-tolerant folks who can eat a substantial amount of starch or sugar and whose blood glucose and insulin barely budge. But take heart: if the exploding popularity of low carb and ketogenic diets is any indication, you're not alone. In fact, there are more of us carb *intolerant* people out there than those whose metabolisms we envy.

We carb intolerants need to be more careful about the types and amounts of carbs we consume. For some of us, when we eat even a relatively small amount of sugar or starch, our insulin rises very high and *stays* high for several hours. Picture the security guard calling for backup and a bunch more security guards coming to stand outside the fat cells and staying there all day long, and you'll have a rough idea of what it's like when we eat more carbs than we can handle. There is *no way* that stored fat is coming out.

Carbohydrate intake isn't the only thing that affects insulin levels but it's the one we have the most control over, so let's focus on that for now. (In chapter 8, we'll look at stress and sleep, which also affect insulin sensitivity and carb tolerance, and might play a role in causing or breaking a fat loss stall.) When insulin is low, fat can be released. (The security guard takes his break.) And the easiest and most effective way to keep insulin low is to keep carb intake low.

This is a key point: when your goal is losing body fat, ketogenic and low carb diets are effective because of the

> When your goal is losing body fat, ketogenic and low-carb diets are effective because of the very low carbs, not because of the high fat, and not because of the ketones.

low carb aspect, not because of the high fat, and not because of the ketones. I don't even like the word "ketogenic" much anymore. It puts the emphasis on the state of ketosis and producing ketones, when this is not the most important aspect of the diet for someone whose goal is fat loss. I also don't like the abbreviation "LCHF," for "low carb, high fat." This gives equal importance to the low carb and the high fat aspects. This works perfectly fine for some people, but not for everyone. When you're aiming to lose body fat and you're having a hard time with it—especially if you're already eating a lot of fat—the "LC" part is more important than the "HF."

One of the most important lessons you can take away from this book is that higher ketones do not cause faster or greater fat loss. Let me say that again: having higher ketones doesn't mean you'll lose more fat or lose it more quickly. Ketones are the *result*, not the cause, of breaking down fat. In fact, it's possible to *gain* body fat while you're in ketosis, and you can lose body fat even if you're not in ketosis. More about this in chapter 5, but for now, don't worry about chasing ketones.

For the purpose of fat loss, what makes keto effective is the absence of carbs, not the presence of tons of fat, nor the presence of ketones. Don't live and die by blood, breath, or urine ketone testing. The people at KetoGains have a fabulous saying that's right on the money: *"Chase results, not ketones."*

Keto is a fat-burning diet, and what helps you burn fat is *not* burning carbs. For most of us, the more carbs we eat, the less fat we burn, so the answer isn't to add more and more fat in order to make meals "more ketogenic," or to use exogenous ketones; the answer is to make sure carbs are always very low.

This is probably pretty different from what you've read or heard from other people about this way of eating. If you're feeling a bit confused, hang tight. I'll cover "fat macros" and fat in general in more detail in chapter 5.

The Macro Myth:
Math, Math, Pain in the Ath

If you've consulted a "macro calculator" online and it hasn't gotten you the results you were hoping for, then you've already discovered that math isn't always the answer.

In case you're brand new to keto and don't know what macros are, "macro" is short for *macronutrient*—protein, fat, and carbohydrate. They're called macros because macro means *large* or *big*. We eat relatively large amounts of protein, fat, and carbs compared to *micronutrients*—micro meaning *small*. Micronutrients are vitamins and minerals, which we consume in teeny, tiny amounts.

Entering your weight and height into a software program and having an algorithm spit out percentages of fat, protein, and carbohydrate for you to aim for is pretty shaky ground to stand on. At the very least, these programs should ask for your body fat percentage, activity level, and maybe even your age. (Evidence suggests most people would benefit from eating more protein as we get older because our bodies don't respond as effectively to the beneficial effects of protein as when we're younger, so we need a bit more to induce those positive aspects.)

I'm not a big fan of *any* macro calculators, but if you really, *really* want to use one—maybe just for a ballpark to start out with—I recommend the one developed by the KetoGains group here: (https://ketogains.com/calculator/#body-composition). The coaches at KetoGains get excellent results, and their calculator is the best one I know of.

Some macro calculators provide you percentages to aim for, for example, 75% fat, 15% protein, and 10% carbs. Sometimes they give you total calories to aim for and/or break this into absolute grams. For example, using the above percentages, if a macro calculator recommends a daily intake of 1600 calories for you, this would be approximately 133 grams of fat (75%), 60 grams of protein (15%), and 40 grams of carbs (10%). This might be exactly the right formula to get you to your goal, *or it might be totally wrong for you.*

Calories and percentages imply that the human body—your wondrous, beautiful, frustrating, infuriating, miraculous, *complex* body—is no more complicated than a dollar store calculator. If this were true, then calorie counting would be a magical solution for fat loss, and the leotard and spandex-clad aerobics craze of the 1980s would have been the end of obesity. If you're reading this specifically because your fat loss is stalled on a low carb or ketogenic diet, though, you'll probably agree with me that it didn't quite work out that way.

It's not that calories *don't matter*; it's that counting them rarely leads to everything magically falling into place. **When you eat the foods that work best for you and avoid the ones that don't, you don't** *have to* **count calories. That's the beauty of this way of eating: you shouldn't** *have to* **turn your meals into calculus assignments.** You know what the meme says: "Ain't nobody got time fo' that!"

If math were the secret to fat loss, you'd already be at your goal weight and you wouldn't be reading this. Many of you have probably already consulted multiple macro calculators, looking for *the one*—the one that would give you the precise amounts of protein, fat, and carbs to eat, and that if you stuck to religiously every day, would work. It would *have to*. Armed with your magic macros, there's no way you *couldn't* lose weight, right?

How's that been working for ya?

If it *hasn't* been working, that tells you that this is not about the math. Or, if it *is* about the math, you have to find the *right* math, and this often looks pretty different from what online calculators suggest for you. Many of them are based on the epilepsy model of keto, with very high fat percentages, moderate-to-low protein, and very low carbs. The very low carbs part is fine; it's the fat and protein recommendations that often lead people astray when their goal is not preventing seizures, but losing body fat. (More on this in chapter 5.) If you decide to check out the KetoGains calculator, (https://ketogains. com/calculator/#body-composition) you might be surprised at how different its recommendations are for you compared to what you were expecting. It will likely suggest more protein and substantially less fat than other calculators you've used. (But I did say they get excellent results!)

> There are many different ways to construct a low carb or ketogenic diet. The one that works best for you might look very different from what you think it's "supposed to" look like.

The point is, if you're trying to lose body fat, don't eat like a person with epilepsy. Fat loss diets and therapeutic diets for serious medical conditions are not the same things. There are many different ways to construct a low carb or ketogenic diet, and some of them—one that works best for you, in fact—might look very different from what you think it's "supposed to" look like.

4
Carb Creep

One of the most common reasons for fat loss stalls on keto is carb creep. All this means is you're eating more carbs than you realize. It's called carb *creep* because it comes on gradually, little by little. It's not diving into a massive pile of pancakes washed down

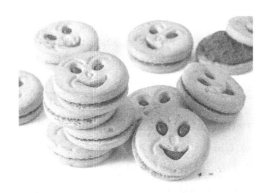

Oh, those sneaky little carbs!

with a glass of orange juice, or a bowl of fettuccini alfredo and bottomless breadsticks. It's a little bit of this, a little bit of that, and just one bite of that other thing—so subtle and slow that you don't even realize it's happening.

If it's happening to you, you might *think* you're very low carb, and compared to what the average person eats, you are, but compared to where *you* need to be in order for *your* body to let go of its excess fat stores, you're a bit too high. (Remember what I said in chapter 2: don't compare yourself to anyone else. If you did well on lots of carbs, you wouldn't be trying keto in the first place.) This is an especially big problem when you're also eating a very high amount of fat—for example, when you're eating a lot of fat, *as if* you were on Atkins induction-like levels of carbs (extremely low, about 20 grams *total* per day), but you're not. You're eating enough carbs to keep you in sugar-burning mode, but since you don't *realize* this, you're combining it with a very high fat intake, *as if* you were a fat-burner (but you're not). So you're burning the carbs and ... storing the fat. For many of us, this high-fat, high-*ish* carb combination is the metabolic kiss of death. It's the standard Western diet that made so many of us sick or overweight in the first place.

To be clear, like I said in chapter 2, everyone's carb tolerance differs. Some people can eat a lot of carbohydrate and still burn plenty of fat because they don't have a large insulin response to the carbs they eat, or their insulin comes back down to a normal level pretty quickly rather than staying elevated for several hours. These are the high-carb tolerant metabolic ninjas we all love to hate. But just because *some* people are metabolically blessed like this doesn't mean we all are. The rest of us have to pull up our big boy shorts and big girl panties and understand that we can't consume as much carbohydrate as we'd like to and still reach our fat loss goals.

Carb creep can come from many different places. For starters, it can come from obvious things, like simply becoming complacent with your diet and consuming things you *know* might interfere with fat loss—foods that are high in sugar or starch and that you're best off avoiding entirely. A slice of bread here, a serving of potatoes there... This is very common: often when we're new to keto, we're excited and motivated and stick strictly to the plan. Over time, though, it's easy to start letting things slide and to become more liberal with carb intake. This

> Combining high-fat with high-ish carbs is the metabolic kiss of death. It's the standard Western diet that made so many of us sick or overweight in the first place.

is especially true if you weren't getting your desired results—if the plan wasn't working, why would you *want* to stick with it? Whatever the reason, understand that you're only human. No guilt, shame, or self-recrimination. Just get right back on the very low carb horse and look forward, not back.

Carb creep can also come from less obvious sources, such as condiments and marinades. When you make things from scratch at home you have total control over the ingredients, but when you dine out or buy packaged sauces and other condiments it can be difficult to tell exactly what's in them. When you shop online or at the store, always read labels and be a carb detective. When dining out, be wary of sauces and dressings described as "glaze" and anything you already know is typically loaded with sugar or corn syrup, like barbecue sauce, ketchup, honey mustard, and sweet salad dressings like French, Russian, Thousand Island, and fruity vinaigrettes. (See Appendix B for the Guide to Dining Out on Keto.)

Sugar alcohols are another major source of carb creep. Food manufacturers aren't blind. Owing to the massive popularity of ketogenic diets right now, they're jumping on the keto bandwagon and are trying to cash in while it's still rolling strong. They're producing bars, shakes, cookies, and other items labeled as being "keto," but with a very high total carb content. This brings us to the issue of net carbs.

Net Carbs

"Net carbs" is the total amount of carbohydrate in a food minus the fiber and sugar alcohols in it. Some people who follow a ketogenic diet choose to count total grams of carbs while others

Counting net carbs gets some people into trouble and you'd be surprised at the difference switching to total carbs can make.

prefer to count net carbs. Using net carbs is a way to be a little more generous with your carb intake while still reaping the benefits of the keto way of eating. For example, subtracting fiber rather than counting total carbs means you can eat a lot more broccoli, spinach, almonds, blackberries, and other higher fiber foods and still stay within your carb limit for the day. However, counting net carbs gets some people into trouble and you'd be surprised at the difference switching to total carbs can make.

Some people who go keto find their sweet tooth disappears quickly and their sugar cravings are gone forever. For others, breaking the sweet habit isn't as easy, and thanks to some very creative food bloggers and cookbook authors, we have more keto dessert and treat recipes than we could make in five lifetimes. Eating a keto cookie, cake, or pie is obviously better than eating the sugar-laden version, but some of us are best advised to avoid even the keto-fied versions, especially the ones you can order online or buy at the store, as opposed to the ones you might make yourself.

The main problems here are sugar alcohols and fiber. Sugar alcohols tend to be bigger culprits than fiber, so let's cover those first.

Sugar Alcohols

You can spot sugar alcohols on food labels by the ending -itol: sorbitol, mannitol, maltitol, xylitol, and erythritol. These give foods a sweet taste but they have a lower glycemic impact than regular sugar—meaning they don't raise your blood glucose or insulin as much as sugar. This is because they're not completely metabolized by the body, so you don't actually *absorb* them fully. In fact, if you've ever overindulged in a bag of sugar-free chocolates sweetened with mannitol, maltitol, xylitol, or sorbitol and found yourself running urgently for the nearest bathroom, you've experienced firsthand the laxative effect these compounds are famous for. Because we don't fully absorb them, they pass through the digestive tract and arrive at the colon, where the bacteria that live there (the "gut flora") feed off of them and ferment them, resulting in gas and loose stools. We in the keto world affectionately call this *"disaster pants,"* and most of us have experienced it. (Consider it a rite of passage—welcome to the club!)

The thing is, just because sugar alcohols have a *lower* glycemic impact than sugar doesn't mean they have *no* impact, and some people are more sensitive to them than others are. For some people, some of these sugar alcohols are almost as bad as regular sugar with regard to blood glucose. Research indicates that erythritol has the lowest effect in most people—no effect in most, in fact. This is why the majority of recipes for keto treats and desserts call for erythritol rather than one of the other sugar alcohols.

For people who are very sensitive to sugar alcohols, consuming too many keto sweets can be a major cause of fat loss stalls. If you think you might fall into this category, I recommend eliminating sugar alcohols from your diet, or at the very least cutting way back if these are a staple of your keto diet. The food purists and keto zealots would burn me at the stake for saying this, but for some people, artificial sweeteners are a better choice. Compared to sugar alcohols, these compounds have almost no impact whatsoever on most people's blood sugar

> Food manufacturers hip to the keto craze are catching on to the net carb concept and are producing items that, on the surface, seem great for keto, but when you dig a little deeper, are loaded with sugar alcohols that might be the reason for someone's stall.

or insulin. Artificial sweeteners include sucralose, aspartame, saccharin, and cyclamate. These are the yellow, blue, and pink packets you see at restaurants and coffee shops, and they're also used in various packaged foods. Brand names you're probably familiar with are Sweet n' Low (saccharin), Splenda (sucralose), NutraSweet (aspartame), and Sugar Twin (cyclamate). These are often found in diet sodas and other diet drinks, such as diet iced teas and sugar-free powdered drink mixes. Many keto-oriented physicians who've made their careers out of helping people lose weight or reverse type 2 diabetes see patients have great success with fat loss and lowering blood sugar while including artificial sweeteners in their diet. The safety concerns over these compounds are largely overblown. If you prefer to err on the side of caution, use stevia instead of artificial sweeteners (there are even stevia-sweetened soft drinks and sodas), but some people find stevia to be bitter and unappealing.

Some of the artificial sweeteners are not suitable for baking with. They either break down chemically when heated or they don't provide the "bulk" some recipes need, and which sugar alcohols typically provide. So if you enjoy keto sweets and treats, you might need to stick with sugar alcohols for those recipes, but if you're also stalled in fat loss, you're better off avoiding those treats altogether for a few weeks to see if that gets things moving again. After all, if what you're doing now isn't working, you've got to *change something*.

To be clear here, sugar alcohols can make ketogenic diets much more enjoyable and easier to stick to for the long term. All I'm saying is that if you're specifically struggling to lose body fat and sugar alcohols are a regular part of your diet, consider eliminating them for a few weeks. If you like to use erythritol in your coffee or tea, a small amount is fine. Mostly what I'm recommending avoiding here is keto bars and other packaged sweet treats that contain large amounts of sugar alcohols, which gives them a low *net* carb count, but a high *total* carb count. Food manufacturers hip to the keto craze are catching on to the net carb concept and are producing items that, on the surface, seem great for keto, but when you dig a little deeper, are loaded with sugar alcohols that might be the reason for someone's stall.

Let's move on to fiber.

Fiber

When people count net carbs, in addition to subtracting sugar alcohols, they subtract fiber. Like I said, food manufacturers know that some of us count net carbs, so they add all kinds of fiber to reduce the net carb content of their products. Fiber, by definition, is indigestible, so if it's not digested, how can it impact blood glucose or get in the way of fat loss?

Evidence suggests that the presence of fiber helps to slow down and possibly reduce the absorption of glucose from food. For example, eating a whole apple would raise blood glucose and insulin less than drinking an equivalent amount of apple juice because the fiber in the apple lessens the impact of the sugar.

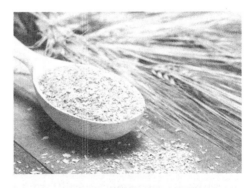

Food manufacturers add this kind of stuff to increase the fiber content of their product so they'll have a lower net carb count. You deserve better than this.

As for something like broccoli, cauliflower, or collard greens, these are very low in carbohydrate to begin with, and we don't digest the fiber, so these have a nearly negligible impact on blood glucose.

Where things get dicey is when products have a high total carb content but a low *net* carb count because of copious added fiber in the form of cellulose, inulin, psyllium, corn fiber, and other fillers. Fiber that's intrinsic to foods—such as that contained in pecans, lettuce, or eggplant, for example—does slow the absorption of carbohydrate and make the total carbohydrate less available to the body (meaning that we don't absorb all of it), but this is not necessarily true for fiber that's added to foods that are high in sugar or starch. Think of it this way: if you added a tablespoon of ground flaxseeds (which are high in fiber) to a large glass of orange juice, do you really think your blood sugar would be all that much lower than if you drank the juice without the flax?

Many packaged bars marketed as "keto" fit this description: 20-25 *total* grams of carbs, but 2-4 grams *net* carbs. Most of the subtraction comes from sugar alcohols, but some of it comes from fiber. As I said, though, this *added* fiber doesn't always have the same effect as fiber that's naturally present in a food, and counting net carbs from these products can be misleading for people who are stuck in a fat loss stall because the fiber isn't having the presumed effect on mitigating the impact on blood glucose and insulin.

Bottom line: if high-fiber packaged products marketed as keto-friendly are a regular part of your diet, consider eliminating them for a while. Consuming higher fiber foods is fine, but stick to foods where the fiber is intrinsically part of the food and is not added as a filler or bulking agent. Think cabbage, lettuce, zucchini, almonds, cucumbers, asparagus, cauliflower, raspberries, avocados, and other naturally fibrous vegetables and fruits.

The Game Plan

Hunker down and get very strict for a few weeks. Approach it like the induction phase of the Atkins diet or Dr. Eric Westman's Page 4 Diet (see Appendix A). Switch from counting net carbs to total carbs and keep it under 20-30 grams *total* per day. Commit to keeping total carbs very low. No swiping onesie-twosies of candy from the dish on a coworker's desk. No small tastes of this or that. Consume keto-friendly foods and keto-friendly foods only, and keep total carbs extremely low. Atkins induction or the Page 4 Diet are arguably the strictest *but most effective* ways to kickstart fat loss, other than straight-up fasting.

Going this low in carbs might mean that you eat fewer vegetables or low-sugar fruits than you were eating before. This is fine. In fact, it's even okay to eat *no* vegetables for a little while and see what happens. There's no such thing as a fiber deficiency. Despite popular conventional belief, you don't need to load up on fiber in order to have normal bowel movements, and some people actually feel *better* with *less* fiber in general or less of certain types of fiber in their diet, particularly if they have digestive issues like bloating, gas, or an irritable bowel condition. Even people with constipation often do better with *less* fiber, not more.[1-5] (If you're already stopped up, why would you want to eat *more* of something intended to "bulk up" your stool?!) There are no essential nutrients you get from plant foods that you can't also get from animal foods, so you're not going to induce any deficiencies in just a matter of weeks if you go to 20-30 total grams of carbs (or fewer!) to see if this gets your fat loss moving again.

If you're currently eating 40-50 grams of

> If you're currently eating 40-50 grams of carbs per day, you'd be surprised at what taking things down to 20 total grams can do. It might sound like a small change, but if you're doing keto and struggling with fat loss, this seemingly small change can make a big difference.

carbs per day, you'd be surprised at what taking things down to 20 grams can do. It might sound like a small change, especially considering it's not unusual for people following a typical Western style diet to consume as many as 200 or 300 grams of carbs in a day, but if you're doing keto and struggling with fat loss, this seemingly small change can make a big difference.

Being this strict with your total carb intake might mean that you have to prepare more of your own food at home. When you cook your own food from scratch, you have total control over the ingredients. If you don't enjoy cooking or you look at your schedule and laugh at the mere thought of having *time* to cook, buying prepared foods is fine, but you'll have to be vigilant about reading labels and buying things you know are definitely suitable for keto. This often means buying *plain* meats and vegetables because seasonings can contain a surprising amount of sugar, corn syrup, corn starch, and other things that can get in the way of fat loss on keto. (See Appendix C for tips on making keto easy when you're on the go or on the road.)

Measuring Ketones

Measuring ketones is not something I normally recommend. In fact, I usually recommend *not* measuring. But if you *think* your carbs are low enough for you to be in ketosis yet you're having a hard time losing fat, maybe they're not as low as you think they are. Testing for ketones in your blood, breath, or urine can show you where you're at, metabolically speaking—specifically, this can tell you if your carb intake is low enough to put you in a fat-burning state.

BUT...

If you're going to test ketones, you need to be aware of a few things so you'll understand how to interpret what you see. I've joked that people should be required to sit through a five-hour biochemistry lecture before being allowed to measure their ketones. If you don't have an appreciation for the spiderweb of different feedback loops and overlapping mechanisms that explain *why*, *how*, and *when* your body produces ketones, you'll drive yourself absolutely crazy wondering why your ketone level isn't what you expect it to be. It's fine to want to measure, but you have to understand how to *interpret* the numbers you see.

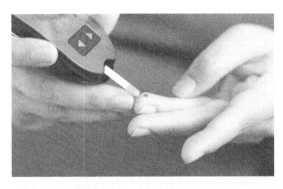

Measuring ketones isn't necessary, but it can be helpful. Whether you measure blood, breath or urine ketones, learn how to understand the results so you don't come to the wrong conclusion.

You can test using whichever method you prefer: urine, blood, or breath. There's some debate about whether the urine test strips are accurate for everyone. Some people claim that they stop working after someone has been keto for a while, but I find this to be untrue for the most part. For most people, the urine test strips work just fine, plus, urine ketone testing is the most economical choice. The strips are relatively inexpensive, and here's a pro tip: cut the strips in half the long way, and you'll have double the strips for the same price. *Score!*

If you test via urine, it's essential to understand that *any* color change is a good sign. You don't have to see dark purple all the time. Even light pink tells you that your body is producing at least *some* ketones, and what *that* tells you is that your insulin is low enough to allow you to burn fat. (Remember the security guard standing outside your fat cells? If you're making *any* ketones, even at a low level, insulin is away on a break.) Seeing the color change—any color change—shows you you're on the right track, which is encouraging and can help you stay motivated to stick with your plan.

Don't test only once a day. Your ketone level naturally fluctuates throughout the day, so if you see light pink first thing in the morning, don't be disappointed. You might see a darker color later in the day, particularly a little while after you've eaten a fatty meal. (But don't get hung up on the color too much anyway; remember that any color change is a good sign.) This is why I suggest cutting the strips in half—if you're going to test a few times a day, it's more economical this way. And remember to give it a few seconds—sometimes the test strips take several seconds to register the full color. If you look at it the instant you pull it away from your urine stream, you might be disappointed, but if you wait 10-15 seconds you'll see a noticeable color change—if you're actually in ketosis, that is.

> It's fine to want to measure, but you have to understand how to *interpret* the numbers you see. If you don't have an appreciation for the spiderweb of different feedback loops and overlapping mechanisms that explain *why, how,* and *when* your body produces ketones, you'll drive yourself crazy wondering why your ketone level isn't what you expect it to be.

Testing ketones via blood or breath is a bit more expensive. Purchasing a breath meter is a larger initial expense but will likely save money over time. Blood meters are inexpensive but the test strips are pricey, making testing multiple times a day cost-prohibitive for most people, unless you have a money tree in your backyard. (If you do, when am I coming to visit?) What I said about urine testing holds true for blood and breath, too: your ketone level naturally fluctuates throughout the day, so don't be disappointed by one reading at one moment in time. Your ketone level might have been higher if you tested an hour before or later. Again, the presence of *any* measurable ketones, even at a low level, means your body is burning fat.

Despite what you might have read far and wide on the interwebs, there's no "threshold" for ketones that guarantees fat loss, or that tells you that you are or are not in ketosis. Some sources say you need to be above 0.5 mmol/L in blood ketones, and some say even higher. Some keto "gurus" out there would have you believe you're not in ketosis unless you're well into 2.0 territory and higher. *This is not true!* If ketones are registering *at all* on your blood meter, congratulations—you're in ketosis. Even something you might think is "too low"—like 0.1 or 0.2 mmol/L— is totally fine and proof that you *are* in ketosis. People's bodies vary in their natural tendency to generate higher ketones. If your level is usually on the low side, that's okay! Plenty of people lose substantial amounts of weight and reverse metabolic illnesses without ever getting into "deep ketosis."

Testing ketones tells you you're burning fat. The thing is, just because you're burning fat doesn't mean you're going to lose body fat. Being in ketosis does not automatically cause fat loss. (Remember

> Testing ketones tells you you're burning fat. The thing is, just because you're burning fat doesn't mean you're going to lose body fat. Being in ketosis does not automatically cause fat loss.

what I said in chapter 3: ketones don't cause fat loss; they're the *result* of breaking down fat.) What measuring ketones does is tell you whether your metabolic state is primed such that you're metabolizing mostly fat and less glucose—that is, whether you're a fat-burner rather than a sugar-burner. This in and of itself doesn't magically lead to fat loss. I know this is confusing, but for now, just know that when your main goal on keto is losing body fat, the best reason to check ketone levels is that if you have measurable ketones in your urine, blood, or breath, even if the level is low, then you know carbs aren't the problem, and this can point you toward another direction to look next with regard to what could be getting in the way of your fat loss. If it's not excess carbs, maybe it's excess fat. Yes, there *is* such a thing as too much fat on keto. We'll get into this in chapter 5.

Let me emphasize again that testing is not essential. I've found it's easy for some people to get carried away with the numbers when they don't even really understand what the numbers mean. The only reason I'm suggesting testing here is because you are specifically struggling with fat loss, and measuring your ketones will tell you whether excessive carb intake is the culprit. And keep in mind that if you choose to test, you don't have to do it forever. Only long enough to get a sense for the types and amounts of food that keep you maintaining a ketogenic state. Once you've established this, you can test once in a while just for fun, or if your fat loss stalls again or you start gaining fat at any point and you want to make sure you haven't strayed too far from what works for you.

What to Do About Carb Creep:

- Consume no more than 20 grams *total* carbs per day, not net, even if this means cutting back on vegetables for a few weeks. (This is a good place to start if you don't want to test ketones: at such a very low level of carb intake, most people will be in ketosis and won't *need* to measure. See Appendix A for the "Page 4 Diet," which gives you instructions for this strict approach.)

- Avoid sugar alcohols unless you know there are certain ones that don't affect your blood glucose or insulin.

- Eliminate keto sweets and treats from your diet. Stick to the basics: meat, poultry, pork, seafood, eggs, cheese, and very low carb non-starchy vegetables. Consider sugar-free jello or 90% cocoa dark chocolate if you must have something sweet.

- Be a label detective: read every label and look for sugar hiding in places you wouldn't expect it. Seeing sugar, honey, or some other caloric sweetener in an ingredient list isn't automatically a deal-breaker. As long as the total carbs per serving fit within your daily carb limit, it's fine. (For example, bacon is often cured with sugar or brown sugar, but the amount remaining in the final product after curing is almost negligible.)

- Cook your own food from scratch as much as possible, or buy prepared foods you're certain are suitable for the strictest form of keto. Dine in restaurants that you trust to prepare your food to your specifications, free of hidden sugars and starches. (See the Guide to Dining Out on Keto in Appendix B for more tips.)

- **No guilt, no shame, no self-blame. Learn from your experience and move forward.**

5
Too Much Fat

Keto is not a license to eat unlimited fat. It's a high-fat diet, but that doesn't mean there are no boundaries, or that you can eat all the fat you like and still lose body fat. It also doesn't mean you need to deliberately add a lot of extra fat to your food, particularly when you're already having a hard time losing body fat. If your

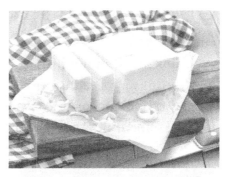

Massive amounts of fat don't make a diet ketogenic; what makes it ketogenic is the absence of carbs.

kitchen sink was backed up, would you add *more* water to it? When there's a traffic jam, the last thing you want is *more cars*.

Here's how keto works: on a high-carb diet, the body's main fuel is glucose (mostly from carbohydrates). When you remove the vast majority of carbs from your diet, your body needs to find some other fuel to use instead, and the fuel it turns to is fat. So when you're in ketosis, or even if you're not actually "in ketosis," but your carbs are low enough that you're primarily running on fat, all that tells you is that you're burning fat. And that's great: the whole point of keto is to switch you from being a sugar-burner to a fat-burner. But what you don't know is whether the fat you're burning is coming from your stored body fat, or from the butter, cream, cheese, nuts, coconut oil, and other fats you're eating. And when you want to lose body fat, you need to *burn* body fat.

Don't add extra fat to things in order to "hit your fat macro." Remember what I said in chapter 3: this way of eating does not work through magical ratios or percentages, so there is *no need* to add extra fat to your meals just to make them line up with a percentage. Adding fat to food doesn't make them "more keto." When your main goal is losing body fat, what makes this diet ketogenic is the absence of carbs, not the presence of copious amounts of fat.

Think about it: if a high fat percentage were responsible for making this way of eating work, then you could eat ten bagels, and as long as you slathered them with enough butter or cream cheese to reach some arbitrary keto ratio or "fat macro," you'd lose weight.

> This way of eating doesn't work through magical ratios or percentages. Adding fat to foods doesn't make them "more keto". When your main goal is losing body fat, what makes this diet ketogenic is the absence of carbs, not the presence of copious amounts of fat.

But that's not how this works. For my Canadian readers— you could eat all the poutine you want and still lose weight. As long as you loaded the fries up with enough cheese curds and gravy to meet your "fat macro" or percentage, body fat would be melting off you.

Keto doesn't work by those kinds of numbers. Remember: *What makes keto effective is the absence of carbs, not the presence of tons of fat.*

"LCHF" or just LC?

I mentioned in a previous chapter that I dislike the abbreviation LCHF because it gives equal emphasis to the low carb and the high fat aspects of this way of eating. That's a great place to start when you're brand new to keto, but once you've made the transition to being a fat-burner, if you're struggling to lose body fat, the high fat aspect becomes a bit less important—and it might even be the culprit behind your fat loss stall.

If your carbs are very low, then insulin will be low. But just because insulin is low doesn't mean you'll magically drop body fat regardless of how much food energy you take in. Even if you're in ketosis, the food energy you take in still has to go somewhere. It has to be used or stored. And if you're going out of your way to load your food up with fat in order to make it "more ketogenic" or to hit some arbitrary macro, you're going to use more of that *dietary* fat, rather than the fat from your hips, belly, thighs, arms, and wherever else you'd like to lose from. After all, that's what stored body fat is *there for:* as an energy supply to be used when there isn't enough energy coming in. If you drink a cup of coffee loaded with 400 calories of butter and coconut oil, your body has no reason to use its backup supply of stored fat.

Hold up a minute...

Am I saying it's all about calories? After so many of us spent decades counting calories and racking up burned calories on treadmills, bikes, or elliptical machines and *failed* to change our physiques, do I have the audacity to say you just need to eat fewer calories?

> Believing that a very high fat intake is the secret to keto is the biggest mistake I see people making with this way of eating when their main goal is fat loss.

No. It's not *all* about calories, but it's maybe a little about them. Contrary to popular opinion, you cannot eat unlimited fat and still lose body fat on a low carb or ketogenic diet. Believing that a very high fat intake is the secret to keto is the single biggest mistake I see people making with this way of eating when their main goal is fat loss. I've even done this, myself, so believe me, I learned the hard way, too. I'm not allowed to keep mayonnaise in my house because my serving size isn't one tablespoon; it's half a jar. And that is *way too much fat* for someone who sits in front of a computer for a living.

Bottom line: the more fat you eat, the less of a need your body has to tap into its stored fat to use for fuel. If you're already lean and happy with your weight, this is no problem. You might *need* a bunch of fat just to maintain your weight. (Lucky you!) But if you're struggling with fat loss on keto despite doing "all the right things," there's a chance you're simply overdoing the dietary fat.

Before moving on, I need to clarify something: everything in this book is intended for people using a ketogenic diet specifically for the purpose of losing body fat. If you're using this way of eating to manage a medical condition that might require a high level of ketones for therapeutic efficacy, that's a different story. There *are* certain situations that might warrant a slightly lower protein intake coupled with much higher fat. But if you're in this for fat loss, that is not *your* situation.

Protein Fearmongering

If you've spent time on ketogenic forums or websites, you've no doubt come across warnings about not consuming too much protein, because...

"It'll turn into sugar!"

"It'll kick you out of ketosis!"

These two phrases need to die a slow and painful death. They represent a total misunderstanding of the biochemical processes at work. Amino acids (from protein) *can* be turned into glucose, but this doesn't happen just because you eat a large chicken breast or go overboard on steak one night. A lesser known fact is that the glycerol portion of triglycerides (triglycerides are the way fats are packaged in foods and also stored in our fat cells) can *also* be converted into glucose, but you

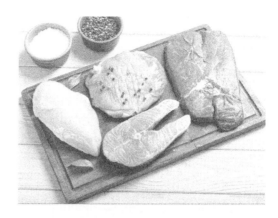

No, these are not the same as chocolate cake. No need to skimp on protein.

never hear anyone saying not to eat too much fat because it'll turn into sugar.

Amino acids *can* be converted into glucose, just like fat *can* be converted into ketones. But neither of these happens just because you eat a lot of protein or fat. They happen under the influence of hormones, mostly insulin and glucagon, but a few others, too. If these things occurred due to mass action—just by loading your body up with them—then you wouldn't need to cut back on carbs *at all* to be in ketosis. You'd just need to consume a ton of fat, because after all, ketones come from fat. But this doesn't happen "just because." It happens because your body's hormonal state *makes* it happen. It's the same with protein: amino acids *can* be converted into glucose, but it

> Amino acids from protein *can* be converted into glucose, but this doesn't happen just because you went wild at the all-you-can-eat meat buffet.

65

doesn't happen in an uncontrolled way just because you indulged at the all-you-can-eat Brazilian churrascaria.

You might have heard that protein affects insulin. This is true, but the effect of protein on insulin is a world apart from the effect *carbs* have on insulin. While we might say that carbs (refined carbs, in particular) *spike* insulin—meaning, they cause a large and very rapid rise, protein induces a gradual, much lower, and *totally physiologically normal* elevation. This is nothing to be afraid of. It's actually a *necessary* effect. In and of itself, insulin is not a bad thing. Insulin is an essential hormone with many critical functions totally unrelated to blood sugar. We need insulin. Too much insulin, too often, is a problem, but we do need *some* insulin. (Too much oxygen or too much water can be deadly, but that doesn't mean we should fear oxygen and water.)

> Eating more protein on a *low carb* diet is very different from eating more protein on a *high* carb diet. The insulin environment is completely different. Most people don't have to worry about eating "too much" protein. In fact, most people could probably benefit from *more* protein, especially if using keto for fat loss.

You probably know that insulin helps gets carbs into muscle cells and certain other cells, but insulin also helps get amino acids into your cells. So if you want to benefit from the protein you're eating—to build muscle, grow your hair and nails, and support maintenance of healthy bones, skin, tendons, ligaments, plus all the *other* stuff made from protein, like antibodies, enzymes, and certain hormones— then you *want* this insulin effect. And I'm using the word "effect" here very deliberately: it's a physiologically normal and necessary effect, not a pathological, harmful "spike."

Beyond that, eating more protein on a *low carb* diet is very different from eating more protein on a *high carb* diet. The insulin environment is completely different, and most people don't have to worry at all about eating "too much" protein. (For a fabulous explanation of this, I recommend the video "Insulin vs. Glucagon: The relevance of dietary protein," from Ben Bikman, PhD.)

In fact, most people could probably benefit from *more* protein, especially if you're using keto for fat loss and even more so if you're having a hard time with that fat loss.

Misguided fear of protein leads people to load up on fat when they're hungry. Instead of having another egg, a can of sardines, tuna, or salmon, or another portion of whatever protein they like (beef, pork, chicken, lamb, turkey...*anything*), they reach for a fat bomb, or put a few spoonfuls of butter or coconut oil in their coffee or tea, hoping the fat will fill them up and tide them over until their next meal.

For some people, this works just fine. Some people do seem to be more satiated by fat than by protein. (Satiation means that you feel full and won't be hungry again for a while.) Others, however, find that protein fills them up better than fat and keeps them feeling satiated longer. If you're one of the people who *doesn't* feel satiated from more fat, you might eat substantially more fat than you need, simply because it's not filling you up and you're afraid to eat protein instead. You think fat is "safe," and you've heard you shouldn't eat too much protein, so you load up on fat but it *still* doesn't satisfy you.

This protein fear has got to go.

The Page 4 Diet and the first phase of the Atkins diet, called "induction"—again, arguably the simplest and most effective ways to get into ketosis and induce fat burning—are *unlimited in protein foods.* Beef, pork, poultry, lamb, wild game, seafood, eggs—*unlimited!* (Now, granted, Dr. Atkins probably said people could eat all they like of these foods under the assumption that no one would eat, say, ten *pounds* of them in a day, so there *is* a limit, but unless someone's paying you to break a world record, most people are in no danger of reaching that limit. Dr. Westman says these foods are unlimited on his Page 4 Diet because he knows that after just a few days, your appetite will be so well controlled that you won't *need* a huge amount to feel satisfied.) These foods are considered unlimited because they're nearly zero carbohydrate and they're very filling and satiating. If someone is having difficulty losing body fat, it's unlikely to be because they're eating too much chicken or bison.

Low Carb High-*ish* Fat

Here are some tips for getting stalled fat loss started again if you think you've been overdoing dietary fat.

Stop drinking liquid calories.

Don't drink liquid fat. You already know drinking liquid sugar (juice, soda, sweet tea) is a bad idea. Heck, even most people *not* on ketogenic diets know soda isn't a health food. (They might be clueless about fruit juice and smoothies, but I digress.) Drinking liquid fat isn't much better when you're having a hard time losing body fat. If you're at your goal physique or are happy with your rate of fat loss, then drink whatever you like, including fat. But if you're reading this specifically because you're struggling, liquid calories should be one of the first things you ditch from your diet. Fatty coffees are the keto equivalent of sugar-sweetened sodas. A small amount of cream in your morning beverage is fine, and even a *small* amount of butter or oil is okay if you really enjoy it, but don't go overboard. If you notice a distinct cognitive or mood boost from MCT oil (which is why most people use it in the morning), then you might want to keep using it and cut a little fat from elsewhere in your diet. But if you don't notice any beneficial effect from fatty beverages and you've been drinking them because you think you're supposed to, or because some out-of-the-box keto program or protocol *told you to*, STOP IT!

If you're having a hard time losing body fat, it's counterproductive to drink a 400-calorie fatty beverage. If you're genuinely hungry, you're better off consuming *actual food*, whether that's a full meal or a small keto snack, like a hard-boiled egg, a can of sardines, pepperoni and cheese, olives, salami, or something like that. And if you're *not* genuinely hungry, *do not add hundreds of calories to your beverage.* Remember the most important thing here: what makes keto work is the absence of carbs, not the presence of and gobs of fat, and having higher ketones doesn't cause faster fat loss, so there's no reason to toss back lots of liquid fat to make yourself "more ketogenic" when you're already having a hard time losing body fat. I know I've said this many times already, and you might be tired of hearing it, but I figure if I say it enough, it'll really sink in.

> What makes keto work is the absence of carbs, not the presence of gobs and gobs of fat, and having higher ketones doesn't cause faster fat loss, so there's zero reason to toss back lots of liquid fat to make yourself "more ketogenic" when you're already having a hard time losing body fat.

Go easy on nuts and cheese.

These are the two most notorious culprits standing in the way of fat loss on keto. To be clear, nuts and cheese are *totally acceptable* on low carb and ketogenic diets. It's not that they're "not keto." The issue is that they are very delicious and *very easy to overeat.* Many of us suffer from "hand to mouth syndrome" when it comes to nuts: You're on the couch or at your desk at work, you've got a bag of almonds or cashews within arm's reach, and before you

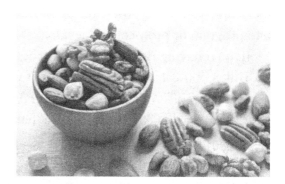

Nuts are fine on keto, but it you know you always overdo them, consider ditching them for a few weeks.

know it, you've blown through half the bag and about 1000 calories with what was supposed to be a snack. The same holds for nut butters. If my mayonnaise problem describes you with nut butters, and your serving of almond or peanut butter is half a jar rather than the 2 tablespoons suggested on the label, it might be best to cut this out of your life for some period of time.

It's the same with cheese. A little bit of cheese is no problem, but many of us sit down with a block of smoked gouda or sharp cheddar and a knife, and it's *game over*. Cheese *gone*. It's okay! No shame! We've all been there. There's no one reading this who can't relate to going overboard with nuts or cheese. Learn from the experience. If you have a hard time controlling yourself with these particular foods, consider eliminating them from your diet altogether, at least for a little while. The nutrient profiles of different cheeses vary, but as a general rule, cheese is higher in protein and slightly lower in fat than nuts are for an equivalent serving size, so if you want to keep some of these very concentrated fat sources in your diet, cheese is probably better than nuts.

Again, the problem isn't these foods, *per se;* it's that most of us overdo them. If you're one of the rare people who *doesn't* lose control with these, and you suspect these aren't the culprits stalling your fat loss, then have at 'em and enjoy.

On the other hand, if you're a mere mortal like most of us, consider eliminating nuts and cheese from your diet altogether for a while. Or if you really want to keep them, use them as a condiment or an addition to a meal rather than a meal or snack by themselves. For example, don't eat nuts as a snack, where you might overdo them. Sprinkle sunflower seeds, slivered almonds, chopped walnuts or pecans onto a salad as a garnish or to add some crunch. Do the same with cheese. Rather than snacking on cheese by itself, top a bunless burger with a slice of cheese or use shredded cheese on a salad or as part of a meal, like a garnish on top of low carb chili, tacos, or steamed vegetables.

Fat bombs—just no

There's nothing wrong with these *if you're at your ideal weight.* But if you've been eating these tasty, very high fat morsels and you're frustrated because your body fat isn't budging, well, I'll leave you to connect the dots here. Fat bombs can be a great tool for people who require high levels of ketones and perhaps even protein restriction for medical reasons. But I find most people eat them for the same reason they drink fatty coffees: because they think they're supposed to, or because they've been scared away from eating more protein. (Or maybe just because they're delicious.) I think I've covered this well enough already. So I'll just leave it at: if you're hungry, eat food—preferably a protein-rich whole food—rather than a concentrated conglomeration of fat.

Trade heavy cream (a.k.a. heavy whipping cream) for light cream or half & half.

This is *total heresy,* I know. If you are really, truly, using only about a tablespoon or two in your coffee (or tea, or wherever else you use it), then heavy cream is fine. But if it's more like 3-4 tablespoons multiple times a day, the fat adds up quickly. If you switch to half & half, there's a very small increase in carbohydrate (about 1 gram per Tbsp) compared to cream, but a large difference in fat. You might also find light cream (sometimes called table cream) at your local store. This is another good swap. It's richer than half & half but not as thick and rich as heavy cream.

Consider using reduced fat cream cheese & sour cream.

Another piece of madness! Maybe not *that* mad, though. If you're struggling terribly with fat loss, you might be better off cutting these things out of your diet entirely, but if you really enjoy dairy and having these things makes keto easier for you to stick to (this is true for many people), then read the labels and see if it would be worth it for you to switch to the reduced fat versions for a while. They often have only 1 or 2g more carbohydrate than the full-fat versions, with significantly less fat. (Some of them don't even have more carbs at all.)

Water down your dressing.

More insanity. Believe me, I know, and I don't enjoy saying this. The whole beauty of keto is that we're *allowed* to eat rich, creamy, high fat foods, right? Yes, this is true. But you're also reading this because you're having a hard time losing body fat, so if you've *already* been loading up on fatty dressings, it probably hasn't been working so well for you. Things like ranch and blue cheese dressing are delicious, and most of us don't really stick to a 2-Tbsp serving. Just like with nuts and cheese, it's easy to go overboard on these very high fat items.

If you absolutely cannot stomach the thought of buying anything with a low fat or "lite" label and you must, *must* have your favorite blue cheese, ranch, caesar or other high-fat dressing, consider thinning it a little with water and vinegar. (Use plain white distilled, apple cider, or champagne vinegar, whatever you like, and whatever works best with that flavor dressing.) This changes the texture a little, yes, but you *do* want to lose body fat, right? Another option is to spend a little extra time at the grocery store and read labels. You'd be surprised at the number of lower fat salad dressings that *aren't* loaded with sugar. An even better option is to make your own, heavy on the vinegar, lighter on the oil. You can make creamy dressings using sour cream or plain yogurt with herbs and spices.

Enjoy your food without added fat.

Just because you *can* add butter, sour cream, mayo, olive oil, and cheese to your food doesn't mean you *have to*. I know I sound like a broken record here, but if you're using this way of eating to lose body fat, then you don't need to add heaps of extra fat in order to make your diet fit special ratios. In fact, doing this might be directly contradictory to your goal. If your steak is already fatty, it doesn't need butter melted on top of it. Don't underestimate the power of salt and pepper. They make almost everything taste better even without any added fat.

Stockpile protein

High-fat items are easy to reach for in a pinch when you're hungry. A bag of nuts, a hunk of cheese, an avocado. Protein can be a bit harder to go for if it's not already prepared and ready to go. Keep a stash of non-perishable protein in your pantry or workplace: canned tuna, salmon, sardines or mackerel, low-sugar beef jerky, or meat-based protein bars. (Always read labels—some contain dried fruit and are surprisingly high in carbs.) At home—or if there's a fridge in your workplace—have a supply of hard-boiled eggs on hand, and embrace eating cold leftover protein. If you're cooking a steak one evening, cook three or four steaks. You can have one for dinner and cut up anther to use in an omelet or salad the next day—or slice it and eat it cold as a snack or quick lunch. The same holds for chicken, pork, or any other protein: cook a large amount at one time; it usually doesn't take any longer than cooking a small amount, and then you'll have plenty left over to grab when you're in a hurry or are hungry and don't feel like cooking.

A slow cooker or pressure cooker is your best friend on keto: you can cook a large piece of meat, like a pork tenderloin or rump roast, with mostly hands-off time, and be able to cut off pieces and eat them cold whenever you're hungry. Lunch meats (cold cuts) are also great to keep on hand. Avoid the obviously higher carb varieties, like "honey baked ham" or "brown sugar turkey," but you'll be able to find plenty of meats that have little to no sugar. Think corned beef, pastrami, and turkey or chicken that's smoked or roasted with herbs. Italian cured meats are great choices for keto: salami, prosciutto, pepperoni, mortadella, etc. Yes, these are a bit higher in fat, but *some* fat is fine! You shouldn't gorge on fat when you're having a hard time losing body fat on keto, but that doesn't mean you have to avoid every last molecule of it, either. (And remember, seeing sugar or some other sweetening agent in an ingredient list doesn't mean the food is off-limits. As long as the total amount of carbohydrate per serving is suitable for you, it's fine. Many lunch meats are cured with sugar, but as is true for bacon, the amount remaining in the final product is very low. Read labels, though, because some *are* too high in carbs.)

Easy Swaps

I've found that for many people—myself included—a lot of extra fat comes in the form of condiments. Salad dressing, mayo, sour cream, etc. The key to keeping things delicious and low carb without racking up a ton of extra fat is to swap out the fattier condiments for things that provide *flavor* without as much fat. Here are some suggestions:

- **Hot sauce:** read labels; you'd be surprised what they sneak sugar and corn syrup into. Sugar isn't necessarily a deal-breaker. Look at the total carb count per serving and be honest with yourself about how many servings you would typically use in a sitting.

- **Pickles/relish:** read labels; some contain sugar or HFCS but most are unsweetened since pickles are intended to be more salty and vinegary rather than sweet. Some brands now have pickles and relish sweetened with sucralose if you prefer a sweet taste.

- **Soy sauce, fish sauce, coconut aminos, or tamari (wheat-free soy sauce):** great for adding salt and flavor, especially to stir-fries or Asian-inspired dishes, like cauliflower fried rice or noodle dishes made with zucchini noodles or shirataki noodles.

- **Salt & pepper:** you'd be amazed at how good these two simple seasonings can make just about anything taste, especially if you use fresh-cracked pepper. Don't be shy with the salt—people on ketogenic diets typically need more salt. Salt is good for you! (The book *The Salt Fix: Why the Experts Got It All Wrong--and How Eating More Might Save Your Life* by Dr. James DiNicolantonio explains this in more detail.)

- **Herbs & spice:** garlic, basil, oregano, rosemary, sage, thyme, dill, curry powder, cumin, cayenne, chili powder, turmeric, cinnamon, parsley, cilantro, etc. – they're all fine!

- **Vinegar:** all varieties are fine, but go easier on balsamic, which is slightly higher in carbs.

- **Homemade vinaigrettes:** heavy on the vinegar, easier on the oil; use mustard or an egg yolk to emulsify/thicken.

- **Fresh-squeezed lemon or lime juice:** in the amount you might use on a salad or squeezed over a grilled chicken breast or piece of fish, the total amount of carbs is almost negligible. (Fresh squeezed lime is highly underrated!)

- **Canned tomatoes:** read labels; many have only 3-5g of carbs per fairly generous 1/2 cup serving, and there are several varieties available, all of which lend a lot of flavor (plain, Italian herb, fire-roasted, green chilies, etc.). Don't bother with any reduced sodium varieties. You *want* the sodium on a low carb diet. Canned tomatoes are great for both sodium and potassium, critical electrolytes on keto.

- **Sugar-free dressings:** There are some pretty good ones available in North America. Maple Grove Farms and Walden Farms are brands that have some good sugar-free flavors, some of which are also low in fat. (Walden Farms are sugar-free and fat-free but contain a litany of ingredients that you might find questionable. If you lean on the side of food purity, you're probably better off making your own dressings anyway.)

What To Do About Excess Dietary Fat:

- Try some of the swaps and substitutions above.

- Bite the bullet and eliminate nuts and/or cheese for a while, especially if you already know they're a problem for you.

- No guilt, no shame, no self-blame. Learn from your experience and move forward.

But Wait!

After all this talk about how to go a bit lower in fat on keto, I have to clear something up so there's no confusion. I'm not trying to make you afraid of fat. Even if you cut back on dietary fat, this is still a high fat diet. If you were eating 70-80% fat and you cut back to, for example, 60%, that's still high fat! And remember, macros and percentages only take into account the food you're eating; they don't include the fat that's coming from your own body. So if you cut back on *dietary* fat and tap a little more into your stored body fat, your body, at the cellular level, is still "eating" a lot of fat. It's just that compared to before, slightly less of that is coming from your plate, and a little more is coming from your hips, thighs, belly, and backside.

If you're aiming for fat loss and the way you've been doing keto so far hasn't been working, think very low carb, higher protein, and lowER fat. This is the approach recommended for people after having bariatric surgery, to help people lose fat and keep it off. It's also an approximation of the diet bodybuilders use to lean out, although they often have to go *really* low fat. If you're not trying to win a professional figure competition anytime soon, you don't have to be quite that austere. You've already mastered the low carb part. To get the stubborn body fat moving, cut back a bit on fat. This doesn't mean you'll be living on grilled tilapia and steamed broccoli, or skinless chicken breast over lettuce. What it means is not chasing arbitrary macros or forcing yourself to eat fat in order to make the math line up.

And you don't want to go super low in fat anyway. You will go stark raving mad if you try. Even when you're trying to lose body fat, you do need some fat coming from your diet for energy, hormone synthesis, optimal nutrient absorption, and not going absolutely loony. So don't be afraid of fat, but don't roll out the red carpet for unlimited entry, either.

6
Low Thyroid Function

If you've taken a detailed look at your diet and in your honest, not-kidding-yourself assessment, excess carbs and fat aren't what's standing in the way of your fat loss, thyroid function is another good place to look. Suboptimal thyroid function is much more common among women than among men, but men aren't immune to it. I've

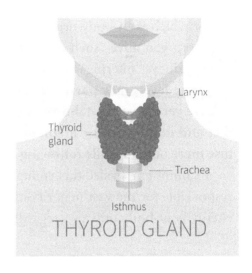

THYROID GLAND

lost count of how many clients I've worked with who had low thyroid function and didn't even know it, or who were actually already on thyroid medication but were not on the right *type* or the right *dose*, so they continued to experience all the signs and symptoms of hypothyroidism—including weight gain or difficulty losing weight.

Role of Thyroid Hormones in Metabolism

Let's start with a brief overview of what the thyroid does. The thyroid gland (which is located at the front of your neck, below the Adam's apple and in front of the windpipe), is often called the "master regulator" of metabolism, owing to its profound influence on how the body uses energy. Healthy thyroid function is crucial for fat loss and weight maintenance, good energy levels, and even a positive mental outlook. **The thyroid helps establish your basal metabolic rate. This is the amount of energy your body uses— the "calories you burn"—while doing absolutely nothing.** It's the rate at which your body uses energy just to run all the processes that keep you alive (such as breathing, your heart beating, and your kidneys filtering your blood). **Differences in thyroid hormone levels may partly account for why some people seem to have very "fast" metabolisms even when they eat a junkfood diet and do no exercise at all, and why others fight like hell to lose mere ounces while following a strict diet and exercise plan.**

I cannot emphasize this enough: your basal metabolic rate is responsible for the vast majority of calories you burn—or, rather, energy your body utilizes—regardless of how much food you eat or how much exercise you do. If your thyroid hormones are out of whack, you will have a very hard time losing body fat no matter how disciplined and diligent you are with regard to diet and exercise. If your body's thermostat is simply set too low, your entire metabolism will be sluggish, *regardless of what you eat and how much you move.* You cannot exercise your way out of a slow metabolic rate due to low thyroid. *You won't burn anywhere near as much energy on a treadmill or in a weight room in 1 or 2 or even 3 hours a day as your body will use all by itself*

> If your thyroid hormones are out of whack, you will have a very hard time losing body fat no matter how disciplined and diligent you are with regard to diet and exercise.

the other 21-23 hours of the day just keeping you alive—assuming your metabolism is not set to super-slow mode.

Owing to its critical role in metabolism and the efficient functioning of many processes in the body, reduced output of thyroid hormone results in an overall slowdown that affects just about everything.

How can you tell if your thyroid hormones aren't at the optimal levels for you? You can have blood tests to measure them and I'll cover that in a bit, but first, let's start with signs and symptoms that can clue you in. It's important to know that you don't have to experience *all* the symptoms below in order to have an underactive thyroid or thyroid hormones that aren't at optimal levels. Hypothyroidism can manifest slightly differently in different people, so if you find yourself saying *yes* to several of the points below, problems with thyroid hormones could be the reason for your fat loss stall, and I recommend getting a comprehensive thyroid assessment. (Details on this in a minute.)

Signs & Symptoms of Low Thyroid:

- Weight gain (or inability to lose weight)
- Hair loss
- Constipation
- Depression; apathy
- Fatigue
- Cold hands and feet; feeling cold all the time
- Dry skin
- Hoarse voice
- Loss of the outer third of the eyebrows
- High cholesterol (total and LDL)
- Low blood pressure
- Slowed heart rate
- Brain fog; cognitive impairment

- Edema (water retention; especially in the lower legs – to the point where your ankles or lower legs look like tree trunks at the end of the day)

Considering the effects of thyroid hormones on metabolism, these signs and symptoms are no surprise. *Everything in the body slows down:* the heart rate, generation of heat, and even the movement of waste through the colon. (Hence the constipation.) Thyroid hormones are required for proper functioning of the LDL receptor, so that's why LDL accumulates in the bloodstream and cholesterol is elevated when thyroid hormones are low.

Low thyroid function doesn't just affect the body; it affects the mind and spirit, too. Many people with hypothyroidism experience depression, so we could say that a sluggish thyroid has physical *and* mental or psychological effects, but depending on how you look at this, mental and psychological effects *are* physical—or, rather, they're biochemical. When someone with hypothyroidism experiences depression, it is not—repeat, *not*— "all in their head." It has its origins in hormonal dysregulation, and telling someone affected by this to "just cheer up" or "look on the bright side" is absolutely not a solution. The depression is driven by an underlying hormonal abnormality that can be corrected. The point is, when thyroid hormones are low, the physical body slows down, but even *thoughts and emotions* slow down. **And you can't talk-therapy your way out of it because these terrible thoughts aren't something you've fabricated for no reason. They're not imaginary. They have a** *biochemical/hormonal* **basis. At best, you can fake it until you (and your doctor)** *actually correct the underlying problem.*

Testing Thyroid Hormones

The most important thing to know is that if you suspect your thyroid is on the fritz, you must ask for a *comprehensive thyroid panel*. You absolutely must insist on this. Thyroid hormone testing is complex and many doctors look at only a fraction of the relevant measurements—a fraction that tells them very little about the overall situation. As a result, countless patients are told their lab values are "normal," yet they will continue to suffer from the sometimes debilitating effects of underactive thyroid. Considering the impact on quality of life when thyroid symptoms are severe, this is truly one of the great medical tragedies of our time. (If this wasn't common as heck, there wouldn't be a book called *Why Do I Still Have Thyroid Symptoms? When My Lab Tests Are Normal* by Datis Kharrazian, PhD, DHSc. Seriously. *Someone wrote an entire book about this*.)

In order to get a complete picture of thyroid function and understand what's really going on, several different hormones must be measured. A proper assessment of thyroid hormones can help guide treatment because there might be a roadblock in a particular pathway, or in some cases the problem isn't with the thyroid gland at all, but somewhere else in the body and the thyroid is simply reacting to that other issue. Measuring only one or two hormones, as many doctors do, is insufficient for uncovering these hidden issues.

A comprehensive thyroid panel should include:

Thyroid stimulating hormone (TSH): TSH is not produced by the thyroid gland itself, but rather, by the pituitary gland (located in the brain). It does exactly what it sounds like it does: it *stimulates the thyroid* to produce its hormones. TSH is often high in individuals with low thyroid function because if the thyroid gland doesn't respond to the "stimulation" by secreting its hormones, more TSH is generated in order to send a more forceful signal. In less common cases of low thyroid function, TSH will be *low*, which means the thyroid gland doesn't receive an adequate stimulus in the first place. Knowing your TSH is important, but it doesn't stand alone. A TSH that's high or low tells you only that TSH is high or low; it doesn't tell you *why*. For that, you need to look at a few other hormones.

Thyroxine (T4): This is the primary hormone produced by the thyroid gland. It consists mainly of the amino acid tyrosine bound to four atoms of iodine. (This is where the "4" in T4 comes from.) T4 is not the most powerful form of thyroid hormone. T4 is secreted into the blood and other tissues must convert it to T3, which is more potent. T4 is measured as *total* T4 (the total amount of T4 in the blood) or *free* T4. Most hormones cannot travel freely in the bloodstream or they would latch on anywhere and wreak all kinds of havoc. Most are attached to a binding protein of some sort, which keeps them inert or inactive until they reach their target tissues. Free T4 is the amount of T4 that is unbound to other molecules and is thus "free" to perform its actions. Low total or free T4 could be a factor in hypothyroidism, and thus, difficulty losing body fat.

Triiodothyronine (T3): T3 is the more potent or "bioactive" form of thyroid hormone. It's responsible for most of the effects we associate with healthy thyroid function and a metabolism that hums along speedily. The thyroid secretes small amounts of T3 but most T3 is produced from T4 in other parts of the body. The enzyme that converts T4 to T3 is called a de-iodinase—it removes one iodine atom from T4, leaving 3. (Hence the "3" in T3. Neat, huh?) This enzyme is selenium-dependent, which is why you might have heard the mineral selenium is important for thyroid function, in addition to the obvious iodine. As with T4, T3 is also measured as total or free T3, with free T3 being a better indicator of thyroid hormone status than total T3.

In my opinion, free T3 is the most telling measurement when

you're experiencing signs of thyroid dysfunction. Other hormones are important too, but believe it or not, many doctors don't measure T3 at all! (Neither total nor free.) They measure TSH only! Their thinking goes like this: if your TSH is normal, then your T3 is probably normal and your thyroid is fine. They assume that if your thyroid *wasn't* fine, your T3 would be low, which would signal the pituitary gland to pump out more TSH. But since the TSH is normal...*Oy!* You can see now why testing only TSH—which, sadly, is very common—is not good enough!

Reverse T3 (rT3): Think of this as a T3 impostor—it fits into the receptor for T3 but doesn't have the same hormonal effect. In fact, it blocks the real T3 from doing its job. (It's considered a "biologically inactive" form of T3.) I wish they would call it impostor T3, because that might help us be more aware of what it does. rT3 is sometimes elevated during periods of heavy stress or a serious illness, as the body's way of conserving energy. Remember, thyroid hormone—free T3, in particular—is responsible for how quickly your body burns through energy. If you're running around doing a million different things at once with no breaks and no downtime, from a biological/evolutionary standpoint, that would be pretty dangerous. So rT3 comes along to *force* you to slow down. Or, rather, since *you* won't slow down, your body will. Your heart will. Your brain will. Your *colon* will. So you'll have a low heart rate. You'll be depressed, cold, constipated, fatigued, and all the other fun stuff that comes along with hypothyroidism. Reverse T3 often goes hand-in-hand with high cortisol. If cortisol is the gas pedal, rT3 is the brake, trying to keep the car (your body) from careening out of control.

Thyroid antibodies: These include thyroid peroxidase (TPO) antibodies and thyroglobulin antibodies (TgAb). Elevations in these indicate an autoimmune attack on the thyroid gland, in which case the underlying problem is not actually in the thyroid, but rather, with an overactive immune system. Autoimmunity that results in hypothyroidism is called Hashimoto's disease, and autoimmunity leading to hyperthyroidism (*over*active thyroid function) is known as Grave's disease.

Thyroglobulin is a kind of proto-thyroid hormone, or a precursor to thyroid hormone. Thyroid peroxidase is an enzyme that attaches iodine atoms to the tyrosine molecules in thyroglobulin, which creates the thyroxine hormone (T4). Antibodies to either of these compounds can mean that you won't produce adequate thyroid hormones. Thyroid peroxidase is a *heme* protein, which means it contains iron. (Like the hemoglobin in your blood.) So adequate iron is necessary for healthy thyroid hormone synthesis. This is one among many reasons why fatigue is a hallmark of iron deficiency anemia.

It seems like whenever people hear about

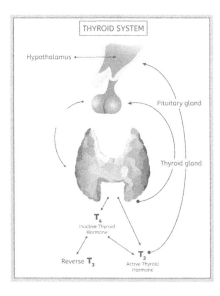

Looking at these images, you can see why testing only TSH or TSH and T4 is often not enough to identify thyroid hormones that are not at optimal levels. And it's not only the thyroid gland itself, where the problem might be, but possibly in the pituitary gland or hypothalamus, which are both located in the brain. It's easier to treat the problem when you know where and/or why the problem is occurring.

hypothyroidism, they assume it's Hashimoto's. "Hashi's" is very common and probably underdiagnosed, but not all thyroid problems are autoimmune in nature. Low thyroid function, or endocrine disturbances elsewhere that affect the thyroid downstream, can happen for a number of reasons, and probably some that haven't even been identified yet.

Bottom line: Measuring TSH alone is nearly worthless. The various thyroid-related hormones are like a Rubik's cube: they interact and influence each other's production, and it's important to look at all of them in order to help things fall into place. (Anyone reading this old enough to remember the Rubik's cube?)

Having a normal TSH does not mean your thyroid is working properly. If your doctor has tested only TSH and told you your thyroid "is fine," yet you *know darn well* you feel awful and are living with multiple signs and symptoms of thyroid dysfunction, you have some options:

1. Politely request that your doctor order a comprehensive thyroid panel.
2. Order one yourself. In the US, you can do this via DirectLabs.com except in Maryland, New Jersey, New York, and Rhode Island. See the note at the end of this chapter for the tests I recommend.
3. *Get a new doctor.* Don't let a well-intentioned but ignorant physician be an obstacle to you reclaiming your quality of life.

Lab Ranges for Thyroid Hormones

Something to keep in mind when assessing your thyroid status is that "normal" is a relative term. Lab ranges differ slightly between testing companies, so what's considered *low* or *high* might be different, too. Depending on the lab used, the very same value could be considered normal or be flagged as out of range. **The**

key is to go by your symptoms. Lab values are a guide and they can help validate or rule out a thyroid problem, but *how you feel* **is much more important. More than the numbers on a lab printout, your signs and symptoms should guide you and your doctor toward the appropriate course of action.**

Far too many people with obvious signs and symptoms of suboptimal thyroid function are told they're "normal" and are provided with no relief. This is partly because some of the signs and symptoms of hypothyroidism are non-specific and can be attributed to other things. For example, weight gain or difficulty losing weight, constipation, fatigue, and depression can be signs of any number of other issues, so thyroid testing isn't always the first place your doctor's mind will go. That being said, as I mentioned earlier, when you have several classic signs of low thyroid, a medical professional ought to at least send you for proper testing. Armed with the results, you'll be able to identify whether you actually *do* have a thyroid problem or rule it out if you don't. Either way, you'll know for certain and can proceed from there more strategically, rather than guessing blindly.

Even though lab ranges are only a guide, here are the basics, with the understanding that you might experience issues related to hypo- or hyperthyroidism *even if you fall within the reference ranges.*

> If you've only had TSH or T4 tested and your doctor said your thyroid is "normal", but you have obvious signs & symptoms of low thyroid, you need better tests...or a new doctor.

Also, as is true for many other measurable biomarkers, conventional allopathic medicine has its preferred ranges, while functional medicine practitioners see things a little differently. You'll notice that some of the ranges overlap, but some have slight differences. Functional medicine practitioners typically interpret lab values with an eye toward what is optimal and will have someone feeling their best, rather than what some random laboratory has deemed "normal." If you experience signs and symptoms of thyroid dysfunction even though your lab values fall within the normal range as defined by conventional medicine, you might find resolution of symptoms by working with a more open-minded doctor who understands the shortcomings of the traditional lab ranges. (The ones here were provided by Justin Marchegiani, DC. Also note that many labs use different units, so if you're comparing your values against these, make sure you're comparing apples to apples.)

If you've been following a solid ketogenic diet without overdoing carbs or fat, and your body fat absolutely isn't budging, *and* you have obvious signs and symptoms of suboptimal thyroid hormone levels, insist on proper comprehensive testing. Don't allow an uninformed medical professional to dismiss your concerns or make you feel like you're imagining everything. (You'd be amazed— or horrified, maybe—at how often this happens. Dealing with a thyroid problem is not for the faint of heart!) Don't let them tell you to eat more fiber for the constipation, or to eat less and move more to get your weight moving, or to give you a statin for the high cholesterol and an antidepressant for your mood. All of these problems are coming from one source, and yes, you might need medication to correct it, but not the medications so many people with hypothyroidism are given to mask the symptoms being caused by the low thyroid hormones. If the thyroid is the problem, then the *thyroid* needs to be addressed. Putting on a sweater because you're cold all the time might warm you up temporarily but it doesn't address the reason *why* you're cold all the time. Laxatives can help you have a bowel movement in the short term, but they do nothing to correct *why* you're chronically constipated. In order to correct the fundamental root cause, you need to address the thyroid, or whatever other endocrine factors are affecting the thyroid.

If you've already had your thyroid tested and were told everything's normal, get a copy of your results and see if a comprehensive testing panel was performed, or if your medical professional is basing her or his evaluation solely on TSH and/or T4. I'm sure it's crystal clear by now that those are not always sufficient.

Test	Conventional Medicine Range		Functional Medicine Range	
TSH	0.27 – 4.20	µIU/mL	1.0 – 2.5	µIU/mL
Total T4	4.5 – 11.7	µg/dL	6.0 – 11.9	µg/dL
Free T4	0.93 – 1.70	ng/dL	1.0 – 1.5	ng/dL
Total T3	80 – 200	ng/dL	100 – 168	ng/dL
Free T3	2.0 – 4.4	pg/mL	3.0 – 4.0	pg/mL
Reverse T3	8 – 24	ng/dL	14.9 – 24.1	ng/dL
TPO Antibodies	<9 – 24	IU/mL	0 – 15	IU/mL
Thyroglobulin Antibodies	≤1 – 24	IU/mL	0.0 – 0.9	IU/mL

Does Keto Affect Thyroid Function?

You might have read some scaremongering pieces online saying that keto is bad for the thyroid, or that people with hypothyroidism shouldn't follow a low carb or ketogenic diet. Neither is accurate.

The truth is, some people with hypothyroid issues find things *improve* when they go low carb or keto. This tends to be more common among people with Hashimoto's than other forms of thyroid dysfunction, but others have reported improvements as well. On the other hand, some people who start off feeling great find that after a while of being keto, they start to have symptoms of low thyroid. What gives? **Is it possible that a way of eating that has such wonderful benefits for so much of the body could be harmful for the thyroid?**

The effect of low carb diets on thyroid function is a controversial issue. Some people following keto find that their T3 decreases after a while. (And remember, T3 is the most active or potent form of thyroid hormone.) At first glance, we might take this to mean that keto causes a slowdown in metabolism, or maybe it has other negative downstream effects. On the other hand, physicians and researchers who've spent decades improving the lives of their patients with low carb and ketogenic diets have not reported adverse effects on thyroid function. So what's the deal?

Well, this is why lab tests are a *guide* and a good starting point, but they shouldn't be the sole arbiter of your health and wellbeing. If your T3 has decreased a bit after you've been following a low carb or ketogenic diet for a while *but you feel fine*, then it's not a problem. In fact, that's true of this entire chapter on thyroid: if you feel well, you probably don't have a thyroid problem. But if you're having a heck of a time losing fat on keto, *and* you're dealing with some of the other signs and symptoms of low thyroid, *then* it's something you should look into.

Back to a lower T3: looked at through the lens of a ketogenic diet, a decrease in T3 doesn't automatically mean your thyroid function is being compromised. In fact, it may be that the improvements in metabolic efficiency people experience while being a fat-burner rather than a sugar-burner result in a heightened sensitivity to T3, and therefore a decreased need for higher levels. That is, their body gets the same effects from a lower level of the hormone. (It's kind of like insulin sensitivity versus insulin resistance: when you are insulin sensitive, you need less of the hormone to provoke its effects than someone who is resistant.) Dr. Stephen Phinney, MD, PhD, who's been doing clinical research on ketogenic diets since the 1980s, has written that this is most likely what's happening, and he's noted that there is no published research showing that well-formulated ketogenic diets induce hypothyroidism. No one really knows for certain what's going on in this situation, though, so this is speculation for now, but it makes sense in light of the physiological mechanisms at work. (You can read Dr. Phinney's article here: www.virtahealth.com/blog/does-your-thyroid-need-dietary-carbohydrates).

What if you've been following a ketogenic or low carb diet, you notice a drop in your T3, and you *do* become symptomatic? This is uncommon, but not unheard of. It's possible this is the result of unintentional caloric restriction. Keto diets tend to induce satiety more easily than high carb diets do—meaning, people feel satiated and stay fuller longer on fewer total calories when they're eating low carb than when they ate high carb. (Not everyone experiences this on keto, but most people do. In fact, not feeling hungry all the time is one of the nicest things about eating this way.) For some people, this increased satiety might mean that, without even trying, they eat a lot less than they did before they switched to low carb. If this happens over the long term, it could affect thyroid function.

But the thing is, *any* diet that results in a very drastic caloric deficit, especially for an extended period of time, would do the same thing. This has been observed in people who lose a lot of weight, especially if it was done through severe calorie restriction. It's called "famine response hypothyroidism."[1-3] In a nutshell, it's a metabolic slowdown in response to drastic energy restriction. Not *carb* restriction, but total food restriction, particularly when combined with a lot of exercise and a generally stressful life.

Remember, your thyroid sets your basal metabolic rate. If you are burning through a lot of energy in a go-go-go lifestyle and doing a lot of exercise on top of that without giving your body the fuel it needs to *get through that,* your body is going take matters into its own hands and correct the situation. You can't go on like that forever or you'll burn out, so as a protective step, you produce less T4 and/or T3, and more reverse T3 – more of the impostor molecule that prevents the real T3 from doing its job. Because you won't slow down and rest or get adequate nutrition voluntarily, your body *forces* you to slow down by making you fatigued, constipated, cold, and depressed. Try hitting the gym when you're fatigued and depressed: your body won't let you. And as for fat loss, well, when your body perceives it's in this crisis, the last thing it's going to do is get rid of its energy reserves. You already don't have enough food coming in; your body's going to conserve the stores it does have rather than burning through them quickly, which would *really* put you into a precarious situation.

Thyroid slowdown, or "famine response hypothyroidism" isn't a unique effect of keto; it's an effect of your body trying to conserve energy because there's been so little of it coming in. When this happens on keto, the assumption is that you need more carbs, or that going so low carb *caused* the thyroid problem. But it's not the lack of *carbs* that did it; it's the lack of adequate total food energy. The solution here isn't necessarily to add back some carbs; the solution is to ensure adequate caloric intake.

A bit of speculation here again, but I suspect unintentional drastic caloric reduction is the culprit behind people becoming symptomatic with regard to low thyroid function on keto. These changes are more common among women than men, and women are more likely to under-consume food energy, whether deliberately or unintentionally. Many women have been living with "diet mentality" for nearly all their lives, and even on a keto diet it can be difficult for them to embrace it being *okay* to eat substantial portions of meat, bacon, cheese, and other fatty foods. They might still be trapped in Lettuce Land, afraid to really let themselves be nourished by adequate amounts of food, particularly when they might have considered these foods "off limits" for most of their life.

Low thyroid function on keto may also be a result of long-term inadequate caloric intake combined with over-exercising. When you work out hard, you have to *rest hard* and *eat hard*, too. Your body needs rest and nutritional replenishment. People who push and push without giving their bodies a chance to rest, repair, and rejuvenate often don't *mean* to do this; it's just that decades of brainwashing have led them to think that 3 ounces of chicken breast and a pile of romaine lettuce is sufficient to "refuel" after an intense workout. So it's not exactly a big shock that they feel better adding sweet potatoes, white rice, or even oatmeal back into their diet.

Maybe it's the carbs, but maybe it's also the calories. Coming from the old diet mentality, some people might feel "safer" incorporating some starches into their diet rather than having a larger steak or an extra pork chop. It's possible someone who thinks keto gave them a thyroid problem would be just fine if they increased their total food intake sticking to low carb foods.

But then again, maybe it *is* the carbs. Some people really, truly, do feel better when they increase their carb intake. I have nothing against that. Not everyone needs to be keto 24/7 to look, feel, and perform their best. Thyroid slowdown on keto tends to occur in people who were already pretty lean and active to begin with— people who didn't need to lose much weight—if any—and who already exercised frequently and intensely. These people likely didn't "need" a ketogenic diet anyway, and simply adopted it to experiment, or because their friends were doing it, or because they were convinced by some social media outlet that keto is the *only way* to go. It's not.

That being said, you're reading this because your fat loss is stalled. Assuming you're still looking to lose a significant amount of fat, you probably *didn't* start keto already being lean and an exercise fiend. So those last couple paragraphs probably don't apply to you, but I had to write them because I know a lot of people worry about these issues, and you might have even seen articles online sounding alarms about keto and thyroid function. People *can* add carbs back to their diet if they feel best that way—some people do. But not everyone *needs* the carbs.

Thyroid Medication

The following is meant only as a general introduction to thyroid medication. A comprehensive discussion of the different kinds of medication and proper dosing is beyond the scope of this book. If you're already taking thyroid medication, this will give you some insights as to whether the type and dose of medication you're taking are optimal for you, and if you're not taking medication but think you probably should be, this can help inform a discussion with your doctor.

There are several different types of thyroid medication, and different ones work best for different people. There's no right or wrong here; there's only *what works for you.*

T4 medications: These medications provide T4 only. Some people do wonderfully on T4-only meds, but remember that your body has to convert T4 into T3. This conversion is impaired in some people, and for them, T4 by itself is not sufficient to resolve thyroid symptoms. I've worked with many clients who were taking T4-only medication and still had every sign and symptom of hypothyroidism they had before the meds. If you are taking a T4-only compound and still feel awful, T4 alone is not enough for you. Testing your total and free T3 levels will tell you whether your body is converting the T4 into T3. (The most common brand name of T4 medication is Synthroid®. Other common brands are TIROSINT® and Levoxyl®. The generic name is levothyroxine.)

T3 medications: These medications provide T3. Since the body gets T3 directly this way, it bypasses problems with the T4 conversion. Since T3 is the more potent form of thyroid hormone, some people feel best when taking T3 in addition to T4. (The most common brand name of T3 medication is Cytomel®. The generic name is liothyronine.)

Natural desiccated thyroid: These medications come from animal thyroid glands, mostly from pigs (porcine). Because they are made from actual thyroid glands, they provide both T4 and T3, plus other thyroid-related compounds not present in synthetic drugs. They are sometimes standardized to contain precise amounts of T4 and T3, but because they come from animal glands and are not synthesized artificially, some brands may have slight variations from lot to lot. Overall, the amount of active hormone in each pill should be similar, though. (There are several different brands available; the most common are Armour® Thyroid and Nature-Throid®)

These compounds go by other brand names outside the US. Regardless of where you live, if you're taking thyroid medication, look up the brand and find out what *type* of medication it is so you'll know if you're on T4, T3, both, or a natural desiccated thyroid product.

Determining the optimal dose can be a long process. Some people feel better quickly on a relatively low dose of medication; others need higher doses that might take time to work up to. If you start with a certain dose but don't feel any better after a few days or weeks, talk to your doctor about trying a higher dose. Don't give up and assume the medication simply doesn't work for you. It sometimes takes a bit of trial and error to identify the right kind of medication and the right dose that will make you come back to life, so be an advocate for your own health and wellbeing.

My Personal Thyroid Story

I speak from experience here. I'm on thyroid medication, myself, after a few years of feeling absolutely *awful*. I had the hair loss, the constipation, weight gain, edema, depression—you name the symptom, I had it. The depression was the worst. At that time, I didn't know as much about all this as I do now. When I first tried thyroid medication, I took it for a full month and felt *no difference*. Zero improvement in any of my symptoms. What I didn't know at the time was that I was taking a very low dose. I trusted the doctor to know what was best for me. Since I didn't know it was a teeny, tiny dose, after the month's supply was gone, I figured the medication wasn't going to help me and I just kind of gave up. BIG MISTAKE!

I suffered through two more years of debilitating symptoms before things became so unmanageable that I decided to try again. I went to a different doctor, one whose approach was very different. This doctor started me on a very low dose, but the difference was, she *told me* it was a low dose, and *explained to me how to find the dose I needed*. She instructed me to take one tablet for 3-4 days, and if I felt no different, to take two. Take two tablets for 3-4 days, and if I felt no different, take three. I was to keep increasing the dose every few days until I felt better. *When I felt well, that was the dose I needed.* What a revelation! Turns out the dose I needed was much, *much* higher than the one I started with, so it's no wonder I felt no better the first time around. I might as well have taken *nothing*.

Even after identifying my optimal dose, things haven't always been easy. Thyroid medication is a bit of a tightrope walk: sometimes I have symptoms of being *over*-medicated, so every now and then I have to reduce my dose a little, and if I feel *low* thyroid symptoms creeping back, I have to bring it back up. It's a balancing act, and I don't always get it right, but in all honesty, my worst day now is better than my best day was before this medication. (If you've never experienced severe chronic constipation, you can't appreciate how magical it is to have regular bowel movements with no pharmaceutical intervention...no laxatives, no magnesium powder, nothing. Just sit down and *go!*)

And I wasn't kidding above when I used the phrase "come back to life." That's what it felt like when the depression lifted: like I had been hibernating, closing myself off from the world in a dark, stuffy room, and someone suddenly turned the lights on and opened a window.

Finding the right type and dose of medication can take time, but know

> Finding the right type and dose of medication can take time, but know that there's hope. If you're dealing with hypothyroidism, you've probably felt awful for a long time. Now at least you know there's a reason why, and there's something you can do about it. There's a light at the end of the tunnel.

that there's hope. If you're dealing with hypothyroidism, you've probably felt awful for a long time. Now at least you know there's a reason why, and there's something you can do about it. There's a light at the end of the tunnel. It might take some time to get there, but you *will* get there.

If you'd like to read the full details of my personal thyroid story, you can find all that here: http://www.tuitnutrition.com/2017/11/thyroid-part3.html

What to Do About Thyroid Function

- If you have signs and symptoms that lead you to suspect you have low thyroid function or a holdup in some other endocrine gland that's affecting your thyroid hormone levels, *get tested!* (Insist on the comprehensive thyroid panel.)

- If your test results indicate that your hormones are not at the optimal levels, work with a doctor to find the right medication and dose for you, or discuss dietary and lifestyle changes that might be effective.

- **No guilt, no shame, no self-blame. Learn from your experience and move forward.**

Additional Thyroid Resources

Thyroid testing from DirectLabs.com*

- Thyroid Panel Complete: includes TSH, total & free T3, reverse T3, total & free T4, T-3 uptake, and free thyroxine index. (This is the one I recommend if you have no reason to suspect your thyroid problem is autoimmune in nature.) (https://www.directlabs.com/TestDetail.aspx?testid=1406)

- Thyroid Panel Complete + Thyroid Antibodies: includes TSH, total & free T3, reverse T3, free T4, thyroid antibodies (TPO and thyroglobulin antibodies), T-3 uptake, and free thyroxine index. (https://www.directlabs.com/TestDetail.aspx?testid=1719)

- Thyroid Panel with TSH plus Free T3 and Free T4: includes TSH, total & free T4, free T3, T-3 uptake, and free thyroxine index. (https://www.directlabs.com/TestDetail.aspx?testid=384)

*Note: I have recommended 3 different tests, but you only need to choose one. The tests are priced differently, so choose the most comprehensive one you can afford.

Books and Websites

The following books and websites can be very educational, but please note that they are not keto-specific.

- The website Stop the Thyroid Madness. An excellent resource for all things thyroid, including proper testing, different medications, and much more. There's also a book by the same name, but the website will be more up-to-date. See the book *Stop the Thyroid Madness* here: https://stopthethyroidmadness.com

  A sequel book called *Stop the Thyroid Madness II: How Thyroid Experts Are Challenging Ineffective Treatments and Improving the Lives of Patients*

- The book *Why Do I Still Have Thyroid Symptoms? When My Lab Tests Are Normal: a Revolutionary Breakthrough in Understanding Hashimoto's Disease and Hypothyroidism*, by Datis Kharrazian, PhD, DHSc. The fact that someone wrote a book specifically addressing people who have hypothyroid symptoms even when their lab tests are "normal" tells you how common this is.

- The book *The Thyroid Connection: Why You Feel Tired, Brain-Fogged, and Overweight -- and How to Get Your Life Back*, by Amy Myers, MD

- The book *Hashimoto's Protocol: A 90-Day Plan for Reversing Thyroid Symptoms and Getting Your Life Back*, by Izabella Wentz, PharmD

7

Medications That Impair Fat Loss

It's incredibly frustrating if your doctor is constantly harping on you to lose weight but they've put you on a medication that's made you *gain* weight or that makes it difficult to lose any. In fact, "frustrating" is probably an understatement. You might feel downright furious, and you have every right to. There are several commonly used medications that cause weight gain or interfere with weight loss. If you're taking one of these, losing body fat will be more difficult for you, even on a strict ketogenic diet.

Medications that come with risk for weight gain are sometimes called "weight-positive" medications. Keto usually decreases the weight gain effects of these medications, but it doesn't make them go away. Weight gain tends to be *less* with these drugs on keto than for someone taking the same drugs and eating a high-carb diet, but "less" weight gain is still weight gain.

"Dr. Google" can be a dangerous minefield to navigate, but if you're taking one or more medications that you think might be interfering with your fat loss, look for information on the side-effects and see if weight gain is among them. Most medications also come with detailed inserts with information about possible side-effects and warnings about adverse events. Most of us discard these papers as soon as we get home from the drugstore without even looking at them, but try to locate yours and actually *read them*. (If you no longer have the inserts, you should be able to get a copy from the pharmacy that filled the prescription.) Even if weight gain or difficulty losing weight aren't listed as side-effects, keep in mind the possibility that medications can have unexpected effects, and they don't happen in everyone the same way. Some people might experience certain side-effects while others don't.

If you're taking a drug known to or suspected to interfere with fat loss, speak with your doctor about possible alternatives. Most conditions have several different kinds of medication to treat them, and if they work through different mechanisms, some might cause weight gain while others don't. See if you can switch from the drug(s) you're taking to one(s) that won't make losing fat so difficult for you.

The Good News

The good news is, several weight-positive medications are taken for conditions that keto typically improves dramatically, and people are often able to discontinue the meds altogether. Examples include insulin injections (for type 2 diabetics, not type 1; people with type 1 will always require at least some insulin), other type 2 diabetes medications, certain heart or cardiovascular drugs, drugs for hypertension (high blood pressure), antidepressants, anti-seizure drugs, pain medication and other anti-inflammatory drugs, corticosteroids (including nasal sprays for allergies), medications for migraines, epilepsy, mood stabilizers, antipsychotics, and more.

Keto is obviously well-known for improving seizure frequency and severity in epilepsy.[1-2] In fact, that's what keto was originally created for—for epilepsy, not for weight loss or diabetes.[3] The past few decades have seen an explosion in research validating the use of low-carb or ketogenic diets for type 2 diabetes and metabolic syndrome, and it's also very helpful for women with PCOS.[4-10] Beyond these conditions, many people find that keto improves mood and emotional stability to the point that they're able to reduce doses or eliminate anti-anxiety, antipsychotic, or antidepressant medications, and keto has also proven beneficial in some cases of bipolar disorder and schizophrenia.[11-15] Keto has also been shown to be beneficial for people with non-alcoholic fatty liver disease (NAFLD), and those who suffer from migraines and acid reflux/GERD.[16-23]

So there's a good chance that keto can help you to stop taking medications that are causing you to gain or hold onto excess body fat. But please, be safe and always work with a physician or other licensed medical professional (such as a nurse practitioner or physician's assistant) who's qualified to help and can guide you in reducing your dose or stopping your medication appropriately and safely. Never adjust or stop medications on your own.

> Work with a physician or other licensed medical professional who's qualified to help and can guide you in tapering down your dose or stopping your medication appropriately and safely. Never adjust or stop medications on your own.

Weight-Positive Medications

The information below on weight-positive medications comes from the Obesity Medicine Association, a professional medical association in the US that formally recognizes low-carb and ketogenic diets as being highly effective for treating obesity.[24]

Condition	Weight Positive or Potentially Weight Positive Medications	
Type 2 Diabetes	Most forms of insulin Sulonylureas Thiazolidinediones Meglitinides	
Hypertension (high blood pressure) or other cardiovascular issues	Propranlol Atenolol Metoprolol Nifedipine	Amiodipine Felodipine Some types of beta-blockers
Epilepsy or other seizure disorders	Carbamazepine Gabapentin Valproate	
Migraine	Amitriptyline Gabapentin	Paroxetine Some types of beta-blockers
Mood Stabilizers	Gabapentin Lithium	Valproate Vigabatrin
Antidepressants	Amitriptyline Imipramine Isocarboxazid Mirtazapine	Doxepin Paroxetine Phenelzine
Antipsychotics	Clozapine Olanzapine Asenapine Paliperidone Quetiapine Sertindole	Lithium Zotepine Chlorpromazine Iloperidone Risperidone
Hypnotics	Diphenhydramine	
Chemotherapies	Tamoxifen Methotrexate Aromatase Inhibitors	Cyclophosphamide 5-fluorouracil Corticosteroids
Hormone Therapy	Glucocorticoids (including nasal sprays Estrogens Progestins (progesterone) - Including implantable or injectable delivery methods, such as hormonal IUD, Depo-Provera® injections, or similar injections Testosterone - however, "T" typically increases lean body mass and reduces fat mass; weight gained is usually not body fat	

Several medications not listed here have variable effects, meaning they might cause weight gain in some people, cause weight loss in others, or have no effect on body weight

What to Do About Weight-Positive Medications

- Research the medications you're taking to see if any of them are known or suspected to cause weight gain or interfere with fat loss.

- If you *are* taking medications that are getting in the way of your fat loss, work with your qualified medical professional to see if you can reduce the dose or switch to a different medication that is not weight-positive.

- **No guilt, no shame, no self-blame. Learn from your experience and move forward.**

8
Sleep and Stress

Two more things that can interfere with fat loss on keto—or any other way of eating—are prolonged stress and insufficient quantity or poor quality sleep. As is true for weight-positive medications, keto can lessen the effects of these issues, but it doesn't make them

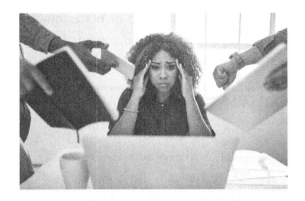

Don't underestimate the effects of chronic stress on your weight and body composition.

go away. To be honest, if your fat loss is stalled on keto, sleep and stress aren't the first places I would look, but that doesn't mean they should be ignored. They don't have as powerful an impact as overdoing carbs or fat does, or as low thyroid function or weight-positive meds do, but they do have an effect.

A strict ketogenic diet will make the effects of these less problematic but they can still get in the way, especially if you're looking to lose just "the last few pounds" and everything else is already dialed in strictly. But don't kid yourself. If you're still eating too much carbohydrate, drowning everything in fat, or you have an uncorrected thyroid problem, lack of sleep probably isn't the main thing standing in the way of your fat loss. So, get all your other ducks in a row, be patient and see if the fat starts moving again, and if not, then take steps to improve your sleep quality and stress management.

Of course, if you'd like to improve those things regardless of your body composition or what you're currently eating, go right ahead! No one's health ever got worse when they were less stressed out and got more sleep or better quality sleep. All I'm saying is, don't expect this to be the magic bullet for breaking your fat loss stall if you know you have other, bigger issues to deal with first.

Stress

When feeling stressed out, some people lose their appetite and don't eat, while others eat *more*. It's interesting that "comfort foods" are typically high in fat, but also almost always high in carbs, too: ice cream, cookies, donuts, potato chips, macaroni & cheese, cupcakes, pizza, french fries, pancakes with butter and syrup. Think about it: even though steaks and scrambled eggs are delicious and satisfying, most of us don't crave them when we're feeling stressed out or overwhelmed.

Emotional and psychological stress affect the entire body. Long-term high levels of psychological stress are associated with increased risk for cardiovascular disease, type 2 diabetes, obesity, depression, and more.[1-9] One of the reasons it's associated with obesity and diabetes is because stress elevates levels of cortisol— one of the hormones responsible for the body's "fight or flight" response.

Cortisol is a "glucocorticoid" hormone. If that word sounds like *glucose* to you, pat yourself on the back; you're exactly right! (It's called a *glucocorticoid* because it affects blood glucose, and it's secreted by the part of the adrenal glands called the cortex.) Cortisol's job is to provide our bodies with glucose in order to help us survive in a life-or-death situation. This glucose is supposed to give us a quick burst of energy to allow us to literally stay and fight, or run (flee) for our lives, hence the aforementioned famous "fight or flight" phrase. (The hormone adrenaline and the neurotransmitter norepinephrine also participate in this.) In the ancient past, this was a great survival mechanism. If you were being chased by a wild animal out on the prairie, you would have needed lots of quick energy to either defend yourself or run away. But in modern times, we almost never face acutely life-threatening situations. More often, we deal with common, everyday stressors that our minds and bodies are hard-wired to *interpret* as immediately dangerous, even though they're far from it.

It's important to note that when I talk about "stress," I'm referring to anything that you perceive as stressful to you, so it doesn't have to be an actual life-or-death emergency. It could be something as simple as being stuck in an aggravating traffic jam, facing a tight deadline at work, or dealing with worrisome financial troubles or a difficult personal relationship. If these types of issues are a constant presence in your life, your blood sugar might be higher than it would otherwise be, even on a low carb or ketogenic diet. And higher blood sugar means higher *insulin*, and higher insulin means difficulty losing body fat.

When you're on a ketogenic diet, the glucose that cortisol puts into the bloodstream doesn't come from dietary carbohydrate; it comes from your own body—from your liver breaking down and releasing stored glycogen, or from turning other compounds into glucose.[10] But don't blame cortisol entirely; this is what cortisol *does*, and it's important. Cortisol isn't the enemy. Just like insulin, the fact that cortisol exists isn't a problem. Too much cortisol, too often, is the problem.

Because of the role of cortisol in raising blood glucose, chronically high levels of stress can be the undoing of the best intentions regarding a low-carb diet. Even if you're eating the right foods and managing your carbohydrate intake, your progress might be stymied by high blood sugar due to stress. Stress won't affect blood sugar and insulin to the same degree that eating, say, a bagel would, but it will affect them somewhat. Your blood sugar might not be sky-high because of stress, but it might be slightly higher than it would otherwise be. And when you're already having a hard time losing body fat, you need every ace you can get.

> Chronically high stress levels can be the undoing of a low-carb diet. Even if you're eating the right foods and managing your carbohydrate intake, high blood sugar from stress could be blocking your progress.

The rise in blood sugar from cortisol wouldn't be much of a problem if stressful situations were rare and resolved themselves quickly. The thing is, some of us feel on edge all day, every day, from the time we wake up until the time we go to sleep. Things seem to come at us from all sides, at all times, both from our external environment and from inside our own heads. *Some* stress is good for us and helps us adapt: "stressing" your heart and skeletal muscles by exercising or lifting weights is painful and damaging in the short term, but it makes those muscles stronger in the long term. But you have to rest and recover between sessions or you'll injure yourself or burn out physically or psychologically. It's the same with mental or emotional stress: you need a break; you can't live it with constantly or it'll wreck you.

Let's be realistic for a moment, though. You might be in a situation where there's very little you can do to reduce your total stress load. Perhaps you're a single parent, a caregiver for an elderly or sick loved one, working two jobs, or are in the midst of some other difficult long-term situation that doesn't exactly give you loads of opportunities for "days off" to relax. Just do the best you can, and *don't be afraid to ask for help.* You might be surprised at how many people in your life would be willing to step up and pitch in once they know you need it.

There are many ways to reduce or relieve stress, and there's no right or wrong way to go about it. The important thing is to *find what works for you.* Common practices for this purpose include yoga, meditation, and deep breathing. If you're not interested in these kinds of pursuits, that's fine. (As they say, one person's pleasure is another's poison. For every person who loves yoga and can't imagine life without it, there's someone like me, who absolutely hates it!) Just make an effort to regularly participate in activities that you do find relaxing. It might be reading, gardening, golf, taking walks in nature, watching comedy movies, photography, knitting, cooking, or something like that. Whatever you enjoy doing and that provides you with relaxation and joy, make a point to have it be a frequent part of your life. Stress reduction can be an important lifestyle factor in improving the disturbed insulin signaling and other metabolic dysfunctions that interfere with fat loss.

The way you respond to stressful situations is entirely under your control. It might not *feel* that way when you're in the middle of something infuriating, but with deliberate intent, you can alter your emotional reactions and mitigate the effects of stress. It's okay—maybe even essential—to unplug now and then. In modern society we tend to celebrate people with "type A" personalities, the ones who are go-go-go, always focused and driven. These aren't *bad* qualities, of course. But the stereotype of an overworked, over-stressed executive (or mom!) who falls ill "all of a sudden" is no coincidence. It's based in a body of truth. People who pride themselves on always being "on," always being reachable, never taking a vacation, eating lunch (and breakfast and dinner!) at their desk, and getting a million and one things done at once do so at significant risk to their long-term physical, mental, and emotional health.

It's okay to take time for yourself. Being selfless and sacrificing your own desires and intentions for the greater good of your family, company, community or other organization are admirable traits, but you don't need to constantly be chasing sainthood for people to love and respect you. By not making time for rest, relaxation, and pursuing some of your own interests, you might be unknowingly standing in the way of your health goals. Contrary to what we tend to believe in the modern industrialized world, disconnecting from work, turning off your phone, hiring a babysitter, taking a vacation, having a "date night," and other ways to stop and catch your breath are not signs of weakness. They're fundamental for good health, and we

> Did you even know you *can* turn your phone off? Yes! There's a power button! You don't have to put it on silent and you don't need an app to block you from using *other* apps. You can turn the darn thing off altogether and forget about it for a while!

dismiss them at our peril. Did you even know you *can* turn your phone off? Yes! There's a power button! You don't have to put it on silent and you don't need an app to block you from using *other* apps; you can turn the darn thing off altogether and forget about it for a while!

I know this can be a tall order for some of you. There are full-time jobs and stressful commutes to contend with, family obligations, and all manner of other commitments. I'm not suggesting that you abdicate all your responsibilities and hop a flight to the closest tropical island without even putting the auto-responder on your email. All I'm saying is, try to find ways, however small or subtle, to reduce your overall stress burden or to help you cope with it better.

Don't dismiss the importance of this. You might be one of the rare people who eats less when they're stressed out, but most of us tend to eat more. And the thing we tend to crave the most is carbs—remember those comfort foods above. The thing is, even if you stay true to keto and don't actually give in to those cravings, the way your hormonal state changes from the stress can cause your body to process the foods you do eat differently. For example, you might have an exaggerated glucose response to your food, or you might secrete more insulin. The exact same foods, in the exact same amounts, can affect you differently depending on your hormonal state at the time you consume and digest them. So even if you eat low carb foods and don't stray from keto, chronic stress can still make fat loss more difficult. And a factor that figures hugely into this is...

Sleep

We all know people who can get by on 4 or 5 hours of sleep and not only do they feel great and look great, but their bloodwork shows that they're in perfect health. However, if you *think* you're getting by on this little sleep but your fat loss is stalled on keto, you're probably not one of those people. (That's a good thing, though; we all hate those people! Or at the very least we're jealous of them. Who *are* these metabolic ninjas, anyway? Part alien?)

Modern industrialized society sometimes feels like a constant competition in which the winners are always doing more: Who can lift the most weight? Who makes the most money? Who drives the most expensive car, or owns the biggest house? There's only one area where people like to brag about how little they do, and that's sleep. It's almost a badge of honor for people to brag about how

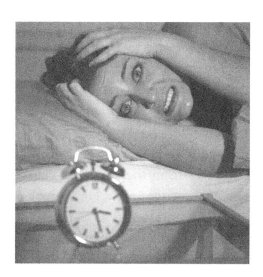

Insufficient sleep or poor quality sleep can interfere with fat loss. Good metabolic things happen when you sleep.

late they stay up, or how little sleep they need to function. (Never mind the coffee they inhale immediately upon waking, or the energy drink they mainline when they start crashing in the late afternoon.) But racking up sleep debt isn't a contest. There's no blue ribbon for winning, and the consequences are no laughing matter. In fact, chronic sleep insufficiency can wreak havoc with metabolism and insulin sensitivity, increasing risk for metabolic syndrome, type 2 diabetes, obesity and other gnarly issues.

Scientists have been researching sleep for decades (at least, maybe centuries) and they're still not sure why we need sleep. We may not know *why* we need it, but we definitely do need it. An absolute requirement for sleep has been identified in every animal species that's been studied. There are no exceptions. We all sleep, and we all *need* sleep. In fact, even *plants* have cycles that can be considered circadian rhythms, mostly based on sunlight and darkness. A detailed discussion of the physiological details of sleep is beyond this book, but there are some important connections between sleep, appetite regulation, hormones, and body composition.

Disruptions in sleep patterns are associated with increased risk for obesity, metabolic syndrome, and other health complications most likely due to the impact of inadequate or broken sleep on insulin sensitivity. Short sleep (not sleeping enough) and broken or fragmented sleep (waking up several times during the night) tend to increase blood glucose response and insulin secretion after meals, as well as result in elevated cortisol levels in the afternoon and evening.[11-16] And these changes can happen after just a few days; they don't take weeks or months to show up. As if all that weren't enough, high cortisol at night can make it difficult to fall asleep ("tired but wired"), creating a vicious cycle of yet more sleep debt and hormonal dysregulation.

> Chronic sleep insufficiency can wreak havoc with metabolism and insulin sensitivity. It increases risk for metabolic syndrome, type 2 diabetes, and obesity. If you're struggling with fat loss, go to *sleep*!

It's telling that the high-stress folks described in the previous section are probably also likely to have chronic sleep debt. Whether they stay up late to get more work done or because they *do* want some time for themselves and long into the wee hours is the only time they can find it, the result is that they might not be getting adequate sleep, and some people live in this pattern for years.

Chronic sleep debt has serious consequences for metabolic

health. Shortened sleep and broken sleep reduce insulin sensitivity and impair glucose tolerance in healthy young people, so the effects might be even more dramatic in people who already have other health problems, and possibly in older people, whose bodies are naturally less resilient.[17,18] Combine this with our natural tendency to seek high-carb foods to provide a quick energy boost when we're tired, and the implications are obvious. A large body of evidence connects chronic short sleep with weight gain and obesity. Weight gain and metabolic rate are influenced by a number of complex biochemical processes that can't be boiled down solely to eating too much and moving too little. However, the conventional advice to "eat less and move more" isn't completely off-base, and insufficient sleep can influence behavior in both of these areas: too little sleep makes us hungry and tired—that is, more likely to eat *more* and move *less*.[15,16] If you're tired and hungry, odds are against you being in the mood to hit the gym.

Weight gain or difficulty losing weight is only one potential consequence of insufficient sleep. Far more nefarious issues can result. For example, due to the role of sleep in regulating insulin signaling and glucose handling, sleep dysregulation is associated with greater risk for type 2 diabetes.[19,20]

Sleep Apnea

Sleep apnea is a huge factor that affects sleep quality and many people aren't even aware they have this condition. Sleep apnea, specifically the variant called *obstructive sleep apnea* (OSA), involves partial or total obstruction of someone's airway so that they experience periodic interruptions in their air supply while they sleep. This lack of oxygen—called *hypoxia*—causes them to wake up several times during the night and also causes dramatic changes to their hormonal profiles, including hormones involved in blood sugar regulation, appetite, the stress response, and the sympathetic nervous system in general.

You might be accustomed to thinking of the stereotypical sleep apnea patient as being overweight or obese. And it's true that many people with sleep apnea are carrying extra weight: the pressure of their own bodies can interfere with keeping their airways open, especially when they sleep on their back. But carrying extra body weight isn't required to have sleep apnea; plenty of people living with OSA are not overweight. Regardless of body weight, OSA is associated with increased risk for type 2 diabetes. One study found that T2D is more prevalent among people with OSA, and people whose OSA was more severe were at higher risk than people with more mild OSA.[23]

Sleep has such a profound impact on blood sugar regulation and the endocrine system as a whole that some researchers believe sleep apnea can be a direct *cause* of insulin resistance or type 2 diabetes.

Obstructive sleep apnea seems to be much more common than we might guess. One study estimated that among the general public, between 4-7% of middle-aged women and 9-14% of middle-aged men are living with moderate to severe OSA, but newer diagnostic criteria suggests the prevalence might be as high as 23% in women and 49% in men.[21] So this isn't an uncommon problem.

How can you tell if you have sleep apnea? Some people are diagnosed through a formal sleep study where they stay overnight at a medical facility and their sleep is monitored. Indirect clues include severe, loud snoring, waking up feeling exhausted, waking up with a sore throat or dry mouth, morning headaches, irritability, forgetfulness, drowsiness while driving, and never feeling rested no matter how much sleep you got—or *think* you got. If there's a partner in your life who shares your bed, they might report that you stop breathing during sleep.

The impact of poor sleep on blood sugar regulation and the endocrine system as a whole is so powerful that some researchers believe sleep apnea can be a direct *cause* of insulin resistance or type 2 diabetes.[22-25] With regard to blood glucose regulation and insulin sensitivity, someone with OSA is probably better off following a ketogenic diet than someone eating a lot of carbs, but even for someone doing keto, their blood glucose and insulin levels might not be quite where we would want them to be because of the interrupted sleep. Remember, even when you eat low carb or keto, your hormonal state has a huge influence over how your body *processes* your low carb foods.

And don't forget, not getting enough sleep is stressful!

Beyond the easily recognizable feelings of anxiousness and irritability we experience when we don't get enough sleep, insufficient sleep is also associated with elevated cortisol levels. This might be another sign of our prehistoric wiring at work: if we're not sleeping enough, perhaps our brains assume there's a reason. Maybe there's a threatening situation going on—a predator nearby, or a conflict with a neighboring tribe—so it's in our best interest to stay awake and remain hyper-vigilant, with cortisol and glucose coursing through our bloodstream keeping us ready to fight or flee at a moment's notice.

Bottom line: don't neglect sufficient sleep. Think of it as Vitamin S—as important and necessary as any other vitamin or mineral.

Beyond the amount of sleep you get, something to be conscious of is your sleep environment. Our hard-wired circadian rhythms expect us to be awake during daylight hours and asleep while it's dark. Lots of artificial light near bedtime and while we sleep can trick our bodies into thinking it's still daytime and as a result we will produce less melatonin—a key hormone that regulates circadian rhythm and helps us fall asleep and stay asleep. Try to remove as much artificial light as possible from your sleeping area. This means no bright digital clocks right near the bed, no streetlight flooding in from outside, and no electronic devices with bright screens just before you go to sleep. If a lot of light from outside comes in through your bedroom windows, consider purchasing "blackout curtains" to make the room you sleep in darker at night. These can be found at most home furnishing stores or ordered online.

You might also consider establishing a routine for "sleep hygiene." In addition to turning off brightly lit electronic devices, this might involve turning the lights down an hour or so before you go to sleep to wind down and ease your body into nighttime. If you're surrounded by bright lights—particularly overhead lights—right up until it's time to get in bed (or possibly even while *in* bed), it'll be difficult for your body to get the signal that it's nighttime and time to go to sleep. (Use table lamps with softer lighting rather than harsh overhead lights if possible. If you have dimmer switches, use them!) You might also consider buying special glasses or goggles that block or reduce blue light (such as from computers or phone screens). Several different brands are available; search for them online, read the reviews, and buy a pair that fits within your budget if you'd like to try these. You can also use apps on your digital gadgets that automatically reduce the blue light they emit or change the color of the screens at a certain time in the evening.

If you have trouble falling asleep, I recommend trying sublingual melatonin lozenges or herbal teas intended to promote restful sleep. Getting sufficient exposure to sunlight during the earlier hours of the day can also help regulate your circadian rhythm and promote better sleep later in the evening.

What to Do About Stress and Sleep

- **Make sure everything else is where it needs to be first:** Make sure your carbohydrate and fat intakes are appropriate for you. Confirm that your thyroid hormone levels are within the appropriate ranges. Check to see if any medications you're taking can cause weight gain or interfere with fat loss, and if so, work with your doctor to find alternatives that don't have this side-effect. Once all of that is taken care of, start prioritizing good quantity and quality sleep.

- **Learn techniques for stress management.** These can be learned from books or apps for meditation, positive affirmations and self-talk, and other helpful strategies. Different things work for different people so it's difficult to make precise recommendations. Find things that work for you, even if they're very different from what works for other people you know personally or people you follow online.

- **Make good quality and quantity sleep a priority.** Easier said than done, I know! This can be difficult for those with large families or who are caregivers for ill or elderly loved ones, so just do the best you can. If you're not able to improve your sleep, it's all the more important to make sure your diet is the best it can be.

- **Get evaluated for sleep apnea if you suspect you have it.** If friends or family complain about your snoring, there's a chance you do. Your doctor can refer you to a sleep clinic for formal testing if warranted. Treatments are available, such as a continuous positive airway pressure (CPAP) machine and other strategies. CPAP machines are not beloved by everyone with OSA. They can be difficult and cumbersome to fall asleep with, but newer models are smaller and quieter than older ones, and compared to increased risk for type 2 diabetes and metabolic syndrome, anything that helps keep your airway open and increases your chances of getting a good night's sleep might be worth trying.

- **No guilt, no shame, no self-blame. Learn from your experience and move forward.**

9
Alcohol Consumption

Can you drink alcohol on keto?

Yes.

Does it interfere with fat loss?

Yes.

My fellow wine, beer, or spirits lovers, rejoice: there *is* room for alcohol on keto. But at the risk of being the bearer of bad news, if you're struggling to lose body fat and alcoholic beverages are a regular part of your life, you can do your fat loss a favor by ditching the booze for a while.

Remember what I said about fatty coffees in chapter 5: when you're having a hard time losing body fat, liquid calories should be the first thing to go. Get your food energy from *food*, not from drinks. And just because many alcoholic beverages are

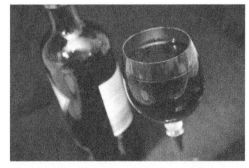

Can you drink alcohol on keto and still lose body fat? Yes, *but...*

low in carbs doesn't mean they're low in calories. It's easy to forget about the calories we drink, but liquid energy can add up quickly, particularly when you're combining it with high-fat meals.

But before everyone has a massive, collective meltdown, let's take a closer look at the issue of alcohol on keto. The truth is, it's best to eliminate it entirely, at least for a while. I'm sorry.

But if that's a total deal-breaker and you're thinking, *"Ain't no way THAT'S gonna happen,"* let's see if there are ways to be more strategic about incorporating alcohol into your life and still get your fat loss moving again.

Alcohol is Burned First

Researchers speculate that our bodies burn different fuels in order of priority, and alcohol is the number one priority. This doesn't mean it's because the body loves it so much that it wants to turn to it first. Mostly it comes down to our storage capacity for different fuels.

Let's look at where the body stores energy, and how much is in each compartment. It helps to think of the body as a hybrid car. We can run on a few different fuels. Unlike a machine, though, the human body is never *on or off, all or nothing*. To some extent, we run on all these different fuels concurrently, but use different amounts in different types of cells and tissues, and depending on various hormone levels.

As you can see below (based on a 155-pound [74 kg] adult), the human body has storage sites—"gas tanks"—for three different fuels: carbohydrate, protein, and fat. That's it. You don't see ketones or alcohol listed as stored fuel types because the body doesn't store them.

Stored Fuel Type	Tissue It's Stored In	Fuel Reserves (grams)	Fuel Reserves (calories)
Protein	Muscle	6000	24,000
Glucose	Body Fluids	20	80
Glycogen (carbs)	Liver	70	280
Glycogen (carbs)	Muscle	120	480
Fat	Adipose (fat cells)	15,000	135,000
Data from: Textbook of Biochemistry with Clinical Correlations, 7th edition. T. Devlin, ed. p.849			

Different fuels the body can run on include:

- Ketones
- Protein
- Carbohydrate
- Fat
- Alcohol

Let's work our way down the list, starting with ketones. Even on a strict ketogenic diet or during a long-term fast, ketones aren't the body's primary fuel. *Fat* is. Fat is used by the majority of the body's tissues except for the few that *can't* use fat. (Yes, there are cells that can't use fat. Fat is burned inside mitochondria, so cells that don't *have* mitochondria, such as red blood cells and certain cells in the retina and adrenal cortex, can't burn them.) On a ketogenic or very low carb diet, ketones can replace glucose as the primary fuel for the *brain*, but not for most of the rest of the body. The rest of the body *can* use ketones, but it uses fats instead, in order to spare the ketones for use by the brain. The brain isn't so great at burning fat, but it's a *champ* at burning ketones, so the rest of the body does it a favor by using fats instead and sending the ketones to the brain.

We don't have anywhere to store ketones, so we metabolize them right away. Some people who use exogenous ketones or MCT oil (which is rapidly converted into ketones) report a rapid increase in energy or a boost in mental clarity and cognition. They feel these effects because ketones are burned quickly. If they weren't, they wouldn't notice these benefits until hours later.

Moving along to protein, even though protein is a source of calories and therefore something we can consider as "fuel," we really don't want to use protein as our main energy source. The example in the table above shows that we have about 6000 grams of body protein, for 24,000 calories of stored fuel. (Protein has 4 calories per gram; 4 x 6000 = 24,000.) Holy moly, that's a lot of stored energy! But *where* is that protein stored? In our muscles, right? And our organs, glands, bones, and other precious tissue that we don't really want to break down for fuel. There's a certain amount of protein "turnover" every day—meaning, old proteins are cannibalized and replaced with new ones, but the old ones still don't come close to being a main fuel source. Amino acids and proteins don't just contribute to the physical structure of muscle tissue. Remember, they're also the raw material for the antibodies your immune system uses to keep you from getting sick, certain hormones (like glucagon and growth hormone), neurotransmitters (like serotonin and dopamine), organs, and blood vessels. Protein is too valuable for these purposes only to have it be siphoned off as an energy source instead. (In the interest of accuracy, there *are* ways in which amino acids from protein are used as fuel, but for the most part, under normal conditions, protein isn't our primary fuel source.) So, bottom line, those 24,000 calories of stored fuel are tempting, but as a main energy source, they're out.

Next down the list is carbohydrate. We often hear that carbs are the body's "preferred fuel." This isn't exactly accurate. It's only true in the sense that carbs (glucose, specifically) will always be used first. Generally speaking, as long as there's a lot of glucose available, the body will use it first instead of turning to some other source of fuel—such as fat, which is why eating a *low carb* diet prompts your body to burn fat instead.

There's really no question that carbs are an energy source, and a quick one, at that. If you've ever fed a toddler a juice box and a couple of cookies and then found yourself having to peel him or her off the walls, that's your proof that carbohydrates are quickly metabolized fuel.

Getting back to the table, our bodies have three compartments to hold carbohydrate (glucose). The first is in body fluids—mostly blood. This accounts for about 20 grams (or 80 calories) of fuel when someone's blood sugar is at a normal level. (A blood glucose of 99 mg/dL [5.5 mmol/L] equates to about 1 teaspoon of sugar in the blood, or 5 grams. The rest of the glucose is accounted for by other body fluids.) If your blood sugar is through the roof, there'd be a lot more than 5 grams in it. 80 calories' worth of fuel? That's not much. In terms of fueling your body, 80 calories is practically nothing, so let's look at the other form of stored carbohydrate in our bodies: glycogen.

Glycogen is to human beings what starch is to plants: it's the form in which we store carbohydrate. Since our blood can only hold so much glucose at any given time (even for a type 2 diabetic with sky-high blood sugar), our bodies have to find somewhere else to stick it. This "somewhere else" is our liver and our muscles. Looking at the table, the liver can only hold about 70 grams of carbohydrate as glycogen, for about 280 calories' worth. That's still not much. As a native New Yorker, I can tell you that just one of those classic New York City bagels nearly the size of your head can pack close to a 70-gram wallop of carbohydrate all by itself. So this liver glycogen, like the glucose in the blood, and like the protein in the muscles, doesn't seem like such a great fuel for the body to rely on.

But the muscles—now we're getting somewhere. Even a relatively non-muscular person has a fair bit of muscle mass. (It might be hiding underneath a thick layer of body fat, but it's still there.) The hypothetical 155-pound person represented in the table stores about 120 grams of carbohydrate in their muscle glycogen, for around 480 calories. Not too shabby, but nothing to brag about, either. If you've ever been to an Italian restaurant in North America, (before your low carb/keto days), you probably crammed more than 120 grams of carbohydrate down the ol' piehole in just one meal. (Breadsticks, pasta, wine, dessert...

heck, you could've gotten 120 grams from dessert *alone*.) 480 calories might sound like a lot, but we're talking about fueling all your muscles, and a basal metabolic rate could easily be 1200 calories—and remember, that's your metabolic rate when you're doing absolutely *nothing*. So, overall, we don't have the capacity to store that much carbohydrate. This might be why carbohydrate appears to be the body's preferred fuel—and I emphasize the word *appears*. Since we can't store a whole lot of it, we *have to* use it first, especially for someone on a high carb diet whose liver and muscle glycogen are already full: it has nowhere else to go.

What about fat? Looking at the table, do you see what I see? This person stores about 15,000 grams of fat in his adipose (fat) tissue, for a whopping 135,000 calories!! *NOW WE'RE TALKING. That* is some serious fuel storage.

The human body has an almost unlimited capacity to store fat and accumulate adipose tissue. Most of us know this only too well: the human body is *great* at socking away extra fuel as fat. And because we can pack away so much of it, we don't need to burn it right away. Why would we burn something we can put away in a nearly unlimited storage tank when we have another fuel—such as carbohydrate—that we *can't* store very much of? As long as there's plenty of carbohydrate—or alcohol—coming in, your body would be silly to burn fat.

Looking at the table, we have no storage capacity for alcohol. None. So when it comes in, we have to do something with it. I know I said our carbohydrate stores are relatively small, but they're not nonexistent. Glycogen stores can be "supersaturated" in some circumstances (like when someone "carb loads" at a pasta party the night before a marathon), and blood glucose can rise very high—as high as 300 or 400 mg/dL (16.6-22.2 mmol/L]) without being acutely life-threatening. An excessively high blood *alcohol* concentration, on the other hand, can be immediately fatal.

Does Alcohol Affect Ketones?

For most people, alcohol doesn't mess much with ketone levels. In fact, for some people, alcohol *increases* ketone levels. It has to do with how alcohol affects the liver, mostly. Your liver normally breaks down its glycogen stores and slowly releases glucose into your blood. Alcohol interferes with this, giving you a lower blood sugar level, and thus, slightly lower insulin and higher ketones. (But

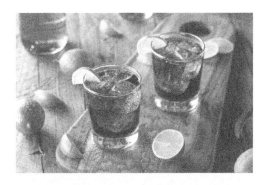

You can drink on keto and still reach your goals if you're strategic about it.

don't use this as a "hack" to raise your ketones! Remember, having higher ketones doesn't cause you to lose body fat faster.)

Medical professionals know that alcoholics often have low HbA1c for this very reason: they run at a lower blood sugar because of their alcohol consumption. Obviously, that doesn't mean they're healthier than someone with a slightly higher A1c. I say again: don't consume alcohol for the purpose of chasing higher ketones.

What to Drink on Keto

Before we talk about which drinks are safest for keto, there's a very important thing you need to know: alcohol hits you *harder and faster* on a ketogenic or low carb diet. You will become intoxicated sooner or on fewer drinks than you might be accustomed to from your high-carb past. No one knows for certain why this happens, but we know it happens. *Pace yourself, and never drink on an empty stomach. Always make sure you are in safe surroundings and have a safe way to get home.*

Also, keep in mind that alcohol lowers inhibitions. When you're drinking, you might be inclined to consume foods you wouldn't normally eat. This might not be true if you're drinking at home and there are no high carb foods available to you, but if you're at a restaurant or a party where sugary and starchy foods are within easy reach, this could spell disaster, especially if you're wired to let one high carb meal or day snowball into several days, weeks or even months off plan.

Okay! Now that that's out of the way, what types of drinks are best for keto?

When you're struggling to lose fat, the best alcohol for keto is *no alcohol*. But I think I've beaten that dead horse enough by now that it's *really* dead. So, with the understanding that you're not going to go the most effective route, let's see how to go the next best way.

For the most part, in terms of carbs, most forms of alcohol are pretty good. Distilled spirits (like vodka, rum, gin, whiskey, bourbon, etc.) actually have *zero carbohydrate*. The problem isn't the spirits, it's what we typically mix them with: orange juice, cranberry or pineapple

> Distilled spirits (like vodka, rum, gin, whiskey, or bourbon) actually have zero carbs. The problem isn't the spirits, it's what we typically mix them with: orange juice, cranberry or pineapple juice, cola, sour mix, etc. Restaurant cocktails and syrupy flavored mixers are typically loaded with sugar.

juice, cola, sour mix, etc. Restaurant cocktails and syrupy flavored mixers are typically loaded with sugar.

With regard to carbs, your best bets are distilled spirits straight-up, on the rocks, or mixed with sugar-free items, like diet sodas, sugar-free tonic water, flavored seltzers, or sugar-free fruit flavored drink mixes or sugar-free cocktail mixers (margarita, cosmopolitan, etc.), which are available online.

Light ("lite") beer is okay, but check the carb count per bottle. Some brands are as low as 2g per bottle, but others are closer to 5g per bottle. That can add up if you're having multiple bottles. (Honestly, though, if you're a true beer aficionado, you're probably better off avoiding beer altogether. Most light beers don't come close to the real thing, and you know this. Save those carbs and calories for something that's *worth it*.)

Wine and Residual Sugar Content

Wine is fine for keto, just avoid the obviously sweet ones. No port, no dessert wines, no ice wines. No sweet Riesling or Moscato. Most people assume red wines are always drier and lower in carbs than whites, but this isn't true. There are sweet reds and dry whites. Even rosé, whose pink

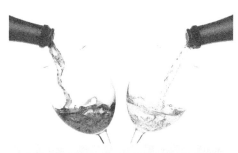

A few companies are marketing "keto wines" now, but you can find perfectly suitable, very low-sugar wines at your local store.

color might make you automatically think it's sweet, can be made very dry. The residual sugar content of wines has more to do with the grape varieties and how the wines are made than with the color.

Residual sugar content of wine varies among brands and vintners—in other words, a cabernet or a chardonnay from one brand might have a different carb count than one from another brand. There are apps that can help you get a general ballpark of the residual sugar content of different wines and even some that can tell you the *exact* sugar content. My recommendation is, if you find a wine you enjoy that you know has a very low sugar content, stick with it.

There are a few companies that now offer wines that are guaranteed to be low in sugar and are marketed as "keto" wines. They're a bit pricier than what you'll find at your local store, but if you want to be absolutely sure you're getting a very low sugar wine and you have the budget for it, purchasing from these companies is a good way to go. Honestly though, you don't have to go out of your way to find special wines. Many brands that you'll see on supermarket shelves or in your state's liquor stores have very little residual sugar and are perfectly fine for keto even though they're not advertised that way. Consider checking out an app that can tell you the sugar content of wines you normally enjoy or ask a store employee to point you toward very low sugar wines. (For that, you might have to go to a specialty wine store; supermarket employees aren't likely to be experts.)

Residual sugar is measured in grams per liter. Here's how to the Liquor Control Board of Ontario (LCBO) classifies wine by sugar content:

Extra dry: 0 - 8 g/L (usually on the lower end; 0 – 4 g/L)
Dry: 3 – 18 g/L
Medium: 18 – 42 g/L
Medium Sweet: 42 – 45 g/L
Sweet: 45+ g/L

Other sources are a bit different:

Dry: 1 – 3 g/L
Off-dry: 10 – 30 g/L
Sweet: > 30g/L
Port/sherry: 50 – 150 g/L
Dessert/ice wine: 100 – 200 g/L

Once you know the amount of sugar per liter, you have some math to do. An entire *bottle* of wine is only 750 mL, so the whole bottle has less sugar than the number given per one liter. And if you're having just one or two glasses, that's even less. So you can see that sticking with dry wines is the way to go: you can have a glass or two for a nearly negligible amount of carbs. (My favorite Malbec has just 2 g/L, so a generous glass is less than 1 gram of carbs. Nice!)

Remember, though, with regard to alcohol, it's not just about the carbs. Even an alcohol that has zero carbs doesn't have zero *calories*. Alcohol falls between fat and carbs in terms of calories: fat has 9 calories per gram, carbs have 4 per gram, and alcohol has 7. Liquid calories don't give you the same satiety as actual *food* that sits in your stomach for a bit, so you might eat the same amount of food and consume energy from alcohol *in addition* to that. If you like to imbibe regularly, think about cutting back on energy from elsewhere in your diet to account for the energy you're drinking.

More Alcohol Resources:

Here are some additional resources to help you make informed choices when looking for alcoholic beverages that can best fit into your ketogenic diet:

- Guide to alcohol on keto from dietdoctor.com, the world's most popular site for ketogenic and low carb diets: Low-carb alcohol – the best and the worst drinks: https://www.dietdoctor.com/low-carb/alcohol

- Handy guide to several wine varieties classified by sweetness, from bone dry to very sweet: Wine Sweetness Chart: https://winefolly.com/tips/wine-sweetness-chart/

To sum up: Alcohol is allowed on keto, but if you consume it regularly and are disappointed with your rate or amount of fat loss, cut out the booze for a while and see if that does the trick.

What to Do About Alcohol

- **Eliminate alcohol from your diet.** I know you don't want to do it, but this is the most effective way to go. Ditch the booze and don't look back.

- **Drink strategically.** If you absolutely, positively will not eliminate alcohol from your diet (and believe me, I understand!), make room for it by cutting back elsewhere in your diet. Alcohol is not calorie-free, so consider reducing fat from somewhere else in your diet to account for the liquid energy you're getting from alcohol.

- **Choose wisely.** Stick to alcoholic beverages that are zero carb or very low in carbs: light beer, dry wine, or distilled spirits. For spirits, drink straight-up or on the rocks, or be sure the mixers you use are sugar-free: diet soda, sugar-free tonic water, sugar-free fruit flavored drink mixes, or sugar-free cocktail mixers (margarita, cosmopolitan, etc.), which are available online.

- **No guilt, no shame, no self-blame. Learn from your experience and move forward.** If you didn't know alcohol could interfere with fat loss, you do now. Proceed accordingly.

10
Exercise

News flash: exercise is not required for fat loss.

I know that probably comes as a shock, but it's true. Or maybe it's not that much of a shock if you're one of the many, *many* people (like me) who dutifully logged hours upon hours on a treadmill, bike, or stair climber, only to see your shape and size stay exactly the same.

What gives? How can someone exercise so much—sometimes multiple hours a day—and not lose fat? Well, remember: high insulin levels get in the way of breaking down fat. So if you were doing a lot of exercise but following a high-carb diet, you were locked in carb burning mode. You might've been desperate to lose weight, and you *thought* you were doing the right thing by avoiding high fat foods. So after a workout, maybe you ate a granola bar, an energy bar, whole grain cereal or something like that—to "refill your glycogen stores," like you probably read about in a fitness magazine. You ate carbs, burned carbs, and refueled or replenished with carbs. Where did *fat* ever enter the picture? It didn't! You were literally

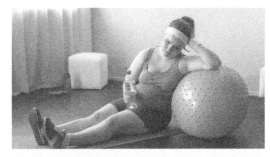

If you've spent years exercising with no change to your size or shape, welcome to the club. Now you know better!

and figuratively on the treadmill to nowhere.

Exercise isn't required for fat loss, and we know this because doctors who use keto in their practices have plenty of success stories from patients who've lost body fat and reversed metabolic disease without exercise. Patients in wheelchairs or who are otherwise disabled have lost body fat and improved metabolic health just fine on keto without pounding the pavement or lifting weights. Also, some people who adopt a ketogenic or low carb diet for fat loss are very, very obese, and it's usually better for them to lose weight *first*, and then add in more physical activity *later*. For someone whose starting weight is very high, intense exercise can put a lot of stress and strain on joints, and some of these folks might also be dealing with fatigue and chronic pain. Someone who's exhausted and whose joints or muscles hurt all the time shouldn't feel like they won't be successful on keto because they can't do a hard workout. Fat loss can definitely come first, and exercise can enter the picture sometime down the line, once they're feeling more energetic. (That's not to say a little walking or something else low-impact, like swimming, can't be helpful, but I'm getting ahead of myself.)

> You ate carbs, burned carbs, and refueled or replenished with carbs. Where did fat ever enter the picture? It didn't! You were literally and figuratively on the treadmill to nowhere.

An interesting study from 2017 compared the effects of a standard American diet (SAD) plus exercise to a ketogenic diet with no exercise, and guess what? Subjects on the ketogenic diet with *no exercise* lost more weight, more *fat*, and had greater improvements in triglycerides and HbA1c than subjects on the SAD with exercise.[1] So, no, if you're on a ketogenic diet, you *don't* have to exercise to lose fat. It's possible the people following the keto diet would have had even better results if exercise *had* been part of the protocol, but the point here is, it wasn't, and they still lost more body fat than the group that exercised. *Diet alone was responsible for the effects seen in the keto group.*

But you don't need me to cite a bunch of nerdy studies on this, right? You've probably lived it. You've experienced it firsthand in your own body. You exercised like a fiend in the past but got nothing for all that effort. And when you switched to keto, some body fat probably came off pretty easily just from the diet alone. But then again, if you're reading this book, it's because your fat loss is stalled or maybe never even got started in the first place. So, what if you're already doing keto but you haven't experienced the magical fat loss everyone else seems to have? *Is* there a role for exercise in this situation?

Exercise isn't a very effective fat loss tool, but that doesn't mean it's totally useless—especially if you're on a low carb or ketogenic diet.

The effect of exercise in people following a low carb or ketogenic diet might be different from the impact of exercise in people eating a high carb diet. Remember what I said earlier: if you're on a high carb diet and you eat carbs, burn carbs, and refuel with carbs, *fat* never enters the picture. On the other hand, if you're on a low carb or keto diet and you're *already burning fat,* then you'll burn proportionally more fat when you exercise.

The human body isn't a binary system. There's no black or white, on

> Even if your weight or size isn't changing, exercise makes good things happen *on the inside.*

139

or off, ones or zeroes. We burn carbs and fat together all the time; it's just that on a high carb diet, we burn a lot more carbs (glucose) and a lot less fat. And we use different fuels when we exercise, too. The intensity of exercise influences which fuel we use more: higher intensity exercise uses more glucose while lower intensity depends more on fat.[2] (You still use some fat during high intensity stuff and some glucose at low intensity, but fat predominates during low intensity and glucose predominates during high intensity.)

If you've ever been near a piece of cardio equipment at a gym, you might have noticed that it had a sticker or a chart on it showing you an age and a heart rate, and whether exercising at a certain percentage of your presumed maximal heart rate put you in the "cardio zone" or the "fat-burning zone." This is laughably oversimplified, but one thing those charts have right is that, generally speaking, when your heart rate is lower and your exercise is less intense, it's likely being fueled more by fat than by carbs (glucose). Another way of saying this is that anaerobic activity is fueled more by carbs, and aerobic activity more by fat. (Aerobic is the stuff you can do for a long time—walking, jogging, even running at a sufficiently slow pace. Anaerobic is the stuff that makes your muscles hurt after just a short time, like lifting weights or sprinting.)

The good news is, when you're on a ketogenic diet and you're mainly a fat-burner, even during high intensity efforts, you'll burn more fat than someone who's on a high carb diet. You'll still use some glucose, but *proportionally*, you'll fuel that high intensity activity with more fat than someone on a high carb diet.[3]

Exercise Versus Burning Calories in Everyday Living

Your body burns calories—*uses energy*—all day, every day, even when you're lounging around doing nothing and even when you're sleeping. It takes a ton of energy just to keep you alive. Breathing, blinking, your heart beating, sitting upright in a chair—all of these things require energy. You don't *feel* like you're burning a lot of energy, but at the cellular level, your body's going through fuel like a champ. (Well, some of us more than others, right? Remember what I said about thyroid hormones: some folks have a fast metabolism while others feel like they're set permanently to slow mode.)

How does exercise fit into this? Not as strongly as you might think.

Let's say you spend an hour at the gym every day. What's more important: the number of calories you burn during that one hour, or what your body is doing metabolically the *other 23 hours of the day*? Let's say you're especially ambitious about losing body fat and you spend *three* hours at the gym. So what? It's *still* more important what your body is doing metabolically the *other 21 hours of the day* than what happens during those 180 minutes of gym time.

Intense exercise can elevate your metabolic rate for an extended period of time afterward—meaning you burn more calories for a while long after your exercise session is over. But this pales in comparison to the amount of energy your body uses daily just to keep you alive. You would have to exercise like crazy to burn through anywhere near the amount of energy your body uses doing almost nothing.

Plus, if you do this too often, for too long, your body will adjust. There's a metabolic adjustment to this amount of physiological stress on your body, the main one of which is a lowering of thyroid hormones. If you work out too hard for too long, for an extended period of time, especially if you combine it with calorie restriction, your body adapts by *slowing your metabolism*. If you watched the show *The Biggest Loser,* you probably know that most of the contestants eventually regained all the weight they lost—and some even ended up with *more* fat than when they started, for this exact reason.[4,5] Your body won't *let you* keep up that kind of exhausting pace while not eating enough. In order to protect you from burning out and completely falling apart, it adjusts your hormones to lower your metabolic rate so you get tired, cold, depressed, and sluggish—you won't *want* to work out when you feel that way. And now that your metabolism is slower, you'll gain weight by eating the *same* amount of food you were eating before. Infuriating!

Don't get caught in this trap. You can lose body fat on keto without exercise.

But...like I said before, just because exercise didn't help you much back in your high carb diet days doesn't mean it's useless. First of all, even if you don't see the scale or tape measure moving, exercise is still good for *health*. It's good for your heart and lungs, good for circulation, and good for *mental health*. While it's not a magic bullet for everyone, many people find that exercise is their best antidepressant.[6,7] For some people, exercise is actually as effective for depression as medication or psychotherapy. What I said about ketogenic diets in chapter 1 applies equally to exercise: even if your weight or size isn't changing, exercise is making good things happen *on the inside*.

Second, now that you're on a low carb or keto diet, the results you get from exercise might be different from what you experienced back in your high carb days. Now that you're *already* a fat-burner thanks to keto keeping your insulin levels low, you'll burn proportionally more fat when you exercise. And if you exercise at a high intensity, you'll go through even more fuel for some period of time after your session is over. The other thing that can be helpful is building muscle from strength training (weightlifting). Generally speaking, the more muscle you have, the higher your metabolic rate will be: it takes energy just to keep that muscle on your body. (There's a reason why professional athletes can eat so much food and not gain weight, and it's not solely due to the amount of time they spend training. They *need* to eat a lot just to maintain their muscle mass.)

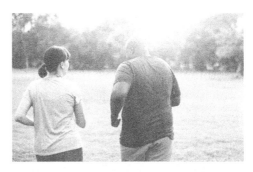

Exercise because you enjoy it and because it does so many great things for your overall physical and mental health--*not because it'll help you lose weight.*

Bottom line: it couldn't hurt to become more physically active. You don't *have to* exercise to lose fat on keto, but it can help. You've probably learned from personal experience (maybe many, many times!) that adding exercise to a high carb diet doesn't usually do much to get body fat moving. But this might not hold true now that you've ditched the carbs. If you're already tackling everything else in this book—carb creep, excess dietary fat, thyroid function, weight-positive meds, stress and sleep, and you live a sedentary lifestyle, consider introducing more physical activity into your life if you can. But if you're unable to do so because of physical limitations, take heart: keto will work for you anyway.

A Note About Exercise and Body Weight

Be aware that if you've been inactive for a long time and you suddenly start an exercise program, you might see your scale weight stay the same for a bit or possibly even go *up* a little. This is especially true if you take up weightlifting. You will be building muscle, so your *weight* might stay the same, but your *shape and size* will change. I can't stress this enough: your *physique* can change substantially even while your *weight* stays exactly the same. (Remember the pictures of Dr. Naiman in chapter 1.) Don't live and die by the scale. As I've explained, scale weight can be very misleading. Use a tape measure or better yet, go by how your clothing fits: your own body will tell you what's happening inside you better than a scale can.

11
Time-restricted eating (TRE), a.k.a. "Intermittent Fasting"

Intermittent fasting is all the rage these days, but I've gotta be honest with you: I don't like this phrase. I like the *concept*, just not the phrase. If you skip a meal or two but are still eating two or even just one meal a

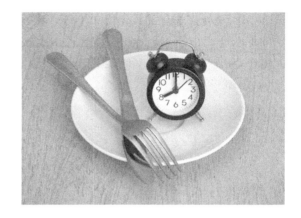

day, is that really fasting? So I'll call it *time-restricted eating*, which better fits what it is: eating your food within a certain number of hours each day and spending some portion of your day *not* eating. It's really just semantics, though. If you like to think of it as intermittent fasting, go right ahead. To*may*to, to*mah*to...in the end, we're talking about the same thing.

Why would anyone deliberately skip meals, or spend 10-18 hours *not* eating? Well, lots of good things happen when you haven't eaten for a while. With regard to fat loss and overall metabolic health, the most important of these is that blood sugar and insulin come down to low-normal levels and *stay there for a while*. Other beneficial hormonal changes happen too, but when you're looking for fat loss, if your insulin is low and it's been several hours since you've eaten a meal, your body will draw from its stored fat in order to fuel itself. You'll also tap into the stored carbohydrate in your liver (glycogen), which is great. (What? Carbohydrate? Yes. Your body and brain do need *some* glucose, but thanks to storing liver glycogen, you don't have to eat bagels and pasta to get it. You can get it from inside your own body, produced on demand.)

The thing is, when you're on a low carb or ketogenic diet, your blood glucose and insulin levels are already low most of the time. Not as low as if you were completely fasting, but certainly lower than back when you were eating a high carb diet. Ketogenic diets induce many of the same beneficial effects seen in fasting even when you don't restrict the total amount of food you eat or the time during which you eat it. Remember that the ketogenic way of eating was originally developed as a medical therapy for epilepsy, because it's been known since ancient times that fasting reduces the frequency and severity of seizures. Once doctors realized that a very low carb, high fat diet "mimicked" this effect of fasting, ketogenic diets became (and still are) a treatment for drug-resistant epilepsy.

> Since eating carbs raises glucose and insulin, by keeping carbs very low, keto keeps glucose and insulin relatively low. And if keeping glucose and insulin low is one of the beneficial effects of fasting, then you're already most of the way there just by eating keto, whether or not you incorporate any fasting.

Since eating carbs raises glucose and insulin, by keeping carbs very low, keto keeps glucose and insulin relatively low. And if keeping glucose and insulin low is one of the beneficial effects of fasting, then you're already most of the way there just by eating keto, whether or not you incorporate any fasting. You're already in a fat-burning state and are burning less sugar. You're already producing ketones (or you will be once you're certain there's no carb creep in your diet). The vast majority of benefits from keto come from a dramatically reduced carb intake and all the good hormonal changes that happen as a result. The question is, are there any *extra* benefits to doing time-restricted eating on top of that? No one seems to know for sure, so for now, my answer to you is a definite maybe.

Why does no one know for sure? The reason is that most of the research in this area has been done in people eating high carb diets! Actually, this is true of *most* health research—on pharmaceutical drugs, surgical procedures, exercise, and pretty much everything else unless a study was specifically looking at effects of lower carb or ketogenic diets. We can't assume that what holds true for someone consuming 45-60% of their calories from carbohydrates would apply equally to someone consuming only 5-10% or even 15-20% of their calories from carbs.

For people consuming a lot of carbs, especially if they eat three meals a day and also snack multiple times a day, it makes sense that they would benefit from a bit of time-restricted eating (TRE). If someone's jacking up their blood glucose and insulin multiple times a day, why *wouldn't* they experience a benefit from taking a break from that and giving those things a chance to come back to normal and stay there for a few hours? (Remember insulin being the security guard that stands outside your fat cells to make sure none of the fat escapes. Only when insulin is lower—such as when you eat much less carbohydrate or you eat *nothing at all*—can that stored fat get out and be burned somewhere else in your body.) But what about someone who's *not* making their glucose and insulin skyrocket most of the day?

If you're specifically having a very hard time losing body fat and you've already got the other things figured out—carbs, fat, medication, thyroid, etc.—there are reasons skipping a meal here and there or eating all your food within a certain period of time and then abstaining for the rest of the day can be helpful even on a ketogenic diet.

Eating anything—including protein or fat—can affect various hormones that influence appetite, satiety, and fuel partitioning (that is, what your body *does* with what you eat). So it's not solely about carbs. People who are very, very insulin resistant or who've been overweight or obese, or have been dealing with severe metabolic problems for a long time might have a higher rise in blood glucose and insulin from a perfectly good ketogenic meal compared to someone who's been slim and healthy all their life. While going strict keto will help these folks a great deal, they might need a little something extra to kick fat loss into high gear if it's stalled.

> If food in general—even low carb food—affects someone's blood glucose or insulin more than normally expected, then it makes sense for them to spend some period of time each day not eating.

This is why snacking isn't such a great idea, especially if you're consuming more carbs than you realize. You might unknowingly be raising your blood sugar or insulin several times during the day. Snacking can work for some people and it's not forbidden on keto, but be careful that your snacks are truly, extremely low in carbs. There are plenty of foods that fit this description, like pepperoni, salami, prosciutto, hard-boiled eggs, pork rinds, or macadamia nuts. But if you're truly hungry, have a meal, and if you're *not* truly hungry, *don't snack.* Snacks are just food that you eat between meals, right? But if you're *between meals,* then you're *between meals,* and hence you should not need to eat.

If you feel hungry between meals, there's a chance your meals are not large enough to keep you satiated for an extended period of time. Consider making your meals more substantial so that you can go a bit longer before feeling hungry again. (I realize there are people for whom this does not apply: for example, if you've had bariatric surgery and physically cannot consume large amounts of food in one sitting, then more frequent smaller meals are appropriate for you. None of this is black & white, my way or the highway. As they say. "Take what you like and leave the rest." Do what's right for you and your particular situation.)

You shouldn't have to force time-restricted eating. Low carb and ketogenic diets are very good at regulating appetite, to the point that you shouldn't feel the *need* to eat or snack around the clock. Three meals a day, or, in some cases, just one or two meals a day, are often enough to keep people satisfied and feeling well physically, mentally, and cognitively, once they're fat- and keto-adapted. If you've been doing keto for a while, you've probably already experienced this firsthand: sure, at some point during the day you feel hungry, but it's not the kind of urgent, immediate, ravenous sense of hunger that comes from wild ups and downs in blood sugar. You feel hungry, but not *hangry*—that crazy combination of hungry and angry most of us know very well.

Like I said above, try not to snack. Eat when you're *hungry,* but make sure you are truly hungry and not just wanting to snack out of boredom or habit, or because you're at a social event and there's food within arm's reach. If you're feeling a little peckish but not genuinely hungry for something substantial, rather than immediately having a snack, wait until you're hungry enough for a full meal.

What About Meal Timing?

Whether you practice TRE or not, does it matter *when* you eat your meals? Should you cut yourself off at a certain time of day? What if you're a shift worker and you *can't* eat at certain times when it's more common for people to eat? (If you're asleep at noon because you work nights, you're not going to wake up just so you can eat at a typical "lunchtime.")

The bottom line on meal timing is: the amount of time you go without food matters more than *when* you eat the food you do eat.

Fortunately, we don't have to go completely by guesswork here. There's been research in this area that can give us some clues as to some of the benefits of TRE and different mealtimes. I have to note, though, like I said above, these studies didn't involve low carb or ketogenic diets, but they still provide us some useful information.

One study involved middle-aged men with obesity who were at risk for type 2 diabetes.[1] The men were instructed to consume their usual diet but were restricted as to *when* they ate: in one part of the study, they ate between 8am and 5pm; in the other part, they ate between 12pm and 9pm. So, both parts had a 9-hour eating window, with 15 hours of "fasting." (They were allowed to consume water, mints, gum, and diet drinks during the fasting hours in order to improve compliance.) The TRE was only done for a week, and even in that short time, there was a major improvement in glucose and insulin response to a test meal after both experiments. Fasting blood glucose levels improved only after the early eating window (8am-5pm), but fasting glucose is a less important measurement than how someone's body responds after a meal, and that's where both TRE interventions showed big improvements. The amount of time spent not eating is what was responsible for the effect, not the timing of when food was consumed.

Not much changed in terms of hormones that affect appetite and fullness, but each part of the study was only one week. Things might have been a bit different if it had been extended for a longer period of time. The fact that there was such a substantial change at all in the glycemic impact of a meal after such a short time—and in people eating their normal diet, not even a low-carb or keto diet—tells us that this is a powerful "hack" that might give you a slight extra edge if your fat loss is well and truly stalled.

Nutrition researcher Alex Leaf wrote an excellent summary of this study, which you can find at https://alexleaf.com/meal-window-not-time-matters-for-health/.

What about eating late at night? If you follow nutrition and health headlines, you've probably heard somewhere along the way that eating late at night is pretty much the worst thing you could possibly do. In the more fanatical circles, eating late at night is practically a sin; people want to burn you at the stake if you admit to doing this. It's probably not the greatest idea to go to sleep with a stomach bursting full of food, but I don't think it's automatically the kiss of death, either.

First of all, some people (me, me!) can't fall asleep if they're hungry. They'll toss and turn with hunger gnawing at them until they get up and head for the fridge. For these folks, having a snack or small meal in the late evening helps ensure falling asleep easily and having restful sleep. For other people, the opposite is true: they can't sleep if they're full. Know thyself, readers: do what's right for you and don't let anyone tell you you're "doing it wrong."

The reason I think it's better not to be completely stuffed when you lie down to get some shuteye is that certain processes are upregulated when we sleep—meaning, they happen more while we're asleep than they do during the day when we're busy running around doing a hundred things. There's something called the *glymphatic system*, which you can think of as the brain's cleaning crew. The glymphatic system helps clear away normal metabolic wastes and other byproducts the brain needs to get rid of, and it's more active during sleep than when we're awake.[2-4]

We don't know for certain, but it's possible that if you eat a large meal right before bed, the hormonal effects of that, and more energy being shunted to your digestive tract, could mean there are fewer resources to devote to the glymphatic system. If your brain "cleans house" best under certain hormonal or metabolic conditions during sleep, and a big meal interferes with those conditions, it's possible you won't experience whatever benefits or possibly even essential functions would otherwise take place. I'm just speculating here, though.

If you're like me and you can't sleep on an empty stomach, I think it's okay to eat at night, especially if it's keto-compliant food. It might not be wise to eat a *huge* meal and then collapse right into bed, but a little bit of something is probably fine. What you eat is more important than when you eat, especially if you're already going several hours without eating during the day.

Fit TRE Around Your Life; Don't Fit Your Life Around TRE.

What works best for your schedule, or for your family dynamic? Some people find it easy to skip breakfast because they're up and out of the house before the rest of the family is even awake. Or they can sit with their family and have a cup of coffee or tea while everyone else eats. If having dinner together as a family or with your spouse or significant other is more important than being together for breakfast, then you might do best skewing your food intake to the later part of the day. On the other hand, if you like starting your day with a meal, do that and skip dinner.

Be flexible. Maybe it's best for you to have a family dinner during the week, but a nice breakfast with your kids on the weekends. Or you like sharing breakfast with your spouse during the week, but you go out for dinner on Saturday nights. If you choose to incorporate TRE into your life, it's entirely customizable—just like keto, itself. *Your* keto diet, and the way *you* implement TRE, could look very different from the way someone else does these things, and you can both get the results you want. Like I said about thyroid medicine: there's no right or wrong here; there's only what works for you.

And be flexible on a daily basis, too. If you normally eat a meal or two early in the day and skip nighttime eating, or you restrict food in the early part of the day and skew your food later, changing this up now and then won't kill you. What if something unexpected comes up and you're not able to consume your meal at the usual time? Maybe an emergency at

> Let your body—not a clock—tell you when to eat. Eat when you feel substantial hunger and don't worry about what time it is.

work pulls you away from your normal mealtime, or you get called for an unexpected social event where it'll look odd if you don't eat anything. It's okay to do things a little earlier or a little later. There is *zero* black and white to this. It's 100% individualizable and you can change it up at any time.

Bottom line: Don't eat by the clock. There's no such thing as breakfast time, lunchtime, or dinnertime. These are artificial constructs mostly built around a traditional office job environment: eat breakfast before you leave for work, eat at mid-day, and then eat again when you get home. But this is totally arbitrary. Let your body—not a clock—tell you when to eat. Eat when you feel substantial hunger and don't worry about what time it is.

Do You *Have to* Fast on Keto?

No! Remember, I wrote this book specifically to help people whose fat loss is stalled. If you're happy with how you look and feel, with your energy levels, your mental clarity, and anything else in terms of your physical and mental health and wellbeing, then keep doing what you're doing. If you're not doing any kind of time-restricted feeding and you feel good, the old saying holds for you: "If it ain't broke, don't fix it."

There was nothing about fasting in the Atkins book. The earliest iterations of low carb and ketogenic diets didn't require fasting. (When ketogenic diets were first used as medical therapy for children with epilepsy, they often started things off with a multi-day fast, but that practice has mostly been abandoned because it's simply not necessary.)

If you look at keto social media these days, it would be easy to think you *have to* fast, or that fasting is a required part of this way of eating. You don't, and it isn't.

You don't have to fast or do any time-restricted eating, but for many people, it happens naturally. Appetite is better regulated, so you don't feel hungry every minute of the day. You can go several hours comfortably between meals and not feel irritable, shaky, tired, or lightheaded. In fact, for some people, lack of intense hunger is an indirect way their body tells them they're either in ketosis or are at least fat-adapted: they can

> You don't have to fast or do any time-restricted eating, but for many people, it happens naturally.

go several hours without eating and without even thinking about food. This is a new world for the many people who always needed to have a snack on hand for "low blood sugar" and for people who couldn't imagine life without snacking all day.

The reason hunger goes away is that you are already eating. Just because you're not putting food into your mouth doesn't mean your *body* isn't eating. You're not consuming food, but your body is, whether it's the food you ate in your previous meal, or glucose being released by your liver and fats being released by your adipose tissue. You're not hungry because now that you're eating keto, your insulin levels are low, which helps you stay a fat-burner rather than a sugar-burner. And since your body can supply itself with fat right from its own stores, *at the cellular level, you are already eating: you're eating your own body fat.*

However, even though you don't *have to* fast or do time-restricted eating, there's a good reason why you might want to:

Resetting Your Relationship with Hunger

Beyond the physical and hormonal benefits that can potentially come from time-restricted eating, perhaps the best reason to incorporate TRE into your life is *psychological*: resetting your relationship with hunger. We're so fortunate to be surrounded by inexpensive and easily accessible food 24/7 that most of us have no idea what it's like to feel true hunger. The second a hunger pang hits, we can reach for a bag or box of something, go to the fridge, or call for takeout...and most of us do. We're uncomfortable with being uncomfortable, and for most of us, hunger is uncomfortable. It's something we want to get rid of as soon as it comes.

But here's the thing: it's okay to feel hungry.

Repeat: It's okay to feel hungry.

You're not actually going to die if you don't eat something the second you start feeling a little peckish. Think about taking a road trip: If you set out on a long car trip and start with a full tank of gas, you wouldn't stop to fill up after driving only one mile, right? Sure, there might be a tiny bit of room in the tank to add a mile's worth of gas, but you'd probably wait until you run through a lot more fuel before topping off. Do the same with your stomach. You don't have to top off at the first sign of there being a little room in there.

Jason Fung, MD, who's been using fasting as a therapeutic tool in his practice for years, makes a great point about hunger. He says it comes in waves. If you get a bit hungry, you don't get hungrier and hungrier and hungrier until you die from hunger or you eat your own hand if there's no food nearby. You do get very hungry, but then it fades. *Ride the wave.* Hunger comes and goes, and it's okay to let it come, power through, and let it go. If you don't snack at the first sign of a hunger pang, you'll be surprised at how much longer you can go without eating.

Wait that out and eat when you are truly, genuinely *hungry—* hungry enough for a meal, rather than picking at something small. If you do find yourself getting hungry between meals, *eat bigger meals.* Maybe your body is present in the here and now, but your *mind* is still living in your low-calorie days, worrying about eating too much, and so you've inadvertently gone too far in the other direction and now you're eating too *little.* If you find yourself genuinely hungry not long after a meal, think about what

> Hunger comes and goes, and it's okay to let it come, power through, and let it go. If you don't snack at the first sign of a hunger pang, you'll be surprised at how much longer you can go without eating.

you ate and ask yourself if it was a substantial enough portion to keep you full for a while. Don't be afraid to eat, especially if you know you have a history of severe caloric restriction or disordered eating. Your idea of what a reasonable, appropriate amount of food is for you might not be accurate.

On the other hand, it's possible you ate a suitable amount of food for yourself, but maybe *what* you ate wasn't the right thing to keep you satiated for long. Maybe there were some hidden carbs in a sauce, condiment, or somewhere else in the meal and you had an unexpected rise and then crash in blood sugar, and it's the low blood sugar causing you to feel hungry rather than a true need for food.

What Can I Consume During a Fast?

This is kind of a funny question, but it's one you'll see on keto social media all the time. If it's "fasting," why do people want to know what they can eat?

Joking aside, there *are* foods and beverages you can consume and still consider yourself to be in a "fasted" state. If you eat or drink anything besides water, I wouldn't consider that truly fasting, but there are certain things you can eat or drink that generally don't interfere with the metabolic effects you're specifically trying to induce through skipping meals or eating within a certain time window, namely, lower blood sugar and insulin, and perhaps enhanced fat burning.

If you'd like to eat or drink certain things during your fasting window, the name of the game is insulin. Stick to things that generally don't affect insulin much, if at all. Why do I keep using the word *generally?* Because there's no black and white here. *Generally* speaking, most people can drink tea or coffee (decaf or regular for both) and not have much effect on their appetite and satiety hormones—or, if anything, the effect in terms of TRE is beneficial: being able to sip on things like that helps people go a bit longer without food. Broth falls into this category, too, whether it's homemade from bones and other gelatinous animal bits or you use bouillon or some other broth base. (Check the ingredients on the label; you never know where they're sneaking in carbs.)

You can add coconut oil or MCT oil to a hot beverage for a ketone boost if you'd like, or a very small amount of heavy cream, and that's okay for most people. Do remember that individual sensitivity varies, though. Munching on a half-ounce of macadamias or walnuts is also a way to extend the time you spend in a semi-fasted state. ("Semi" because the nuts have calories, of course, but they have a negligible effect on blood glucose and insulin, and in the context of being the only things you consume over a period of several hours, you'll still reap the metabolic benefits of TRE.)

If you were using fasting as a therapeutic strategy for a specific medical condition (under physician supervision only, please), my advice would be different. There might be reason to avoid even things that are pure fat if someone is fasting as a medical therapy. But if your main purpose in implementing a TRE strategy is losing body fat or simply maintaining metabolic health, small amounts of these things should be no problem.

To learn more about benefits of TRE and different ways to implement it, the best resource I know of is Dr. Ted Naiman's guide to intermittent fasting...and it's free! To get it, visit https://www.dietdoctor.com/intermittent-fasting/time-restricted-eating.

You can watch a video I did about meal timing on keto on YouTube: "Meal Timing on Keto" by Tuit Nutrition.

12
Take an Information Vacation

Keto rules your life. You eat, sleep, and breathe keto, keto, keto, and you're still not getting the results you want. You read every blog, listen to every podcast, watch every video, subscribe to every newsletter, and you

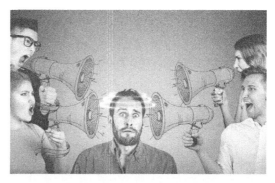

Conflicting information coming at you from all sides? Stop listening for a few days.

post on every forum and support group, and You. Are. About. To. Rip. Your. Hair. Out.

When all else fails...

Take a break!

It's okay to not think about keto 24/7. In fact, it's probably *good* for your mental and emotional health to step away for a few days. Obsessing over it like crazy hasn't helped you so far, so why keep doing it? *STOP!*

If you spend all day every day immersing yourself in all things keto and your frustration has you two seconds away from chucking everything and diving head-first into a half-gallon of ice cream, *STEP AWAY FROM THE KETO.*

I don't mean step away from *eating* keto. I mean step away from the endless amount of confusing, conflicting, and contradictory information. This way of eating is supposed to make your life better, not worse. Easier, not harder, and simpler, not more difficult. If you find your mental health going in the opposite direction—you're anxious, fearful, worried, and every brain cell you have is occupied with thinking about macros, insulin, ketones, autophagy, and your weight—*take an information vacation.*

If your life revolves around weighing and measuring your food, tracking your heart rate, your sleep, your bowel movements, your ketone level, your blood glucose, your workouts, the number of steps you take in a day, and more, and you feel like if you let up for even one second, the entire edifice you're propping up is going to come crashing down around you, this chapter is for you.

If diving down every keto rabbit hole you find has become your main hobby, I totally understand. Perhaps, like me, you spent years doing what you thought were "all the right things" to get healthy or improve your physique. And, perhaps, like me, after years—decades, maybe—of that *failing* you, you discovered the world of carbohydrate restriction, and after learning nearly all the health and fitness beliefs you once held dear were false, you now have a desire—no, an obsession—to learn as much as you can, as fast as you can, from as many different sources as you can. No one could blame you! You've got years of misinformation to correct, right? Nearly a lifetime of programming to de-program.

However, do any of the following describe you with regard to keto?

- Overwhelmed
- Demoralized
- Discouraged
- Frustrated
- Disappointed
- Confused
- Overwhelmed

No, you're not imagining things. I put *overwhelmed* on the list twice, because you're probably feeling overwhelmed enough that it *deserves* to be listed twice. It probably doesn't make you feel any better, but you're not alone. Do you think I would've written this book if I thought there was only one person out there who could be helped by it? I wrote it because I hear from people multiple times a week who are stressed out and feeling boxed in by the emotions above. I even started a YouTube channel to help people understand how truly simple this is when you brush aside all

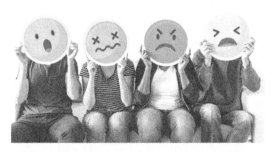

The internet gets ugly sometimes. It's okay to step away for a little while.

that's not necessary to make it work. My motto there is *"Keto Without the Crazy."*™

If the emails I receive from confused and overwhelmed people are any indication, a lot of you out there are afflicted with what's called "paralysis by analysis." The uncertainty, anxiety, and darn near anguish people feel over this stuff are palpable. *I can feel them radiating out of the emails.*

I'm not one to name names, so to keep things friendly, feel free to fill in the blanks with whichever keto personalities make this flow best for you (even if one of them is me!).

_____ said on his podcast last week...

But then _____ wrote on her blog the week before, that...

And that totally contradicts what _____ said in their YouTube video last month...

And in _____'s book, she said that's not how it works, and...

_____ tweeted something completely different, but...

I saw _____ speak at the low carb conference last year, and he said...

No wonder so many of you have whiplash. You'd be a ninja if your neck *wasn't* injured by now. And I have to admit that I often feel this way, myself. If you think my education in nutrition stopped when I graduated, think again. Not only do I constantly read the new (and not-so-new) scientific literature on topics of interest to me, but I also read the same books and blogs, listen to the same podcasts, and watch the same videos you do. I, too, get confused. I, too, feel overwhelmed. So I know of what I speak here.

What is an Information Vacation?

Simple. It's a few days, maybe even a week, where you stay away from keto and low carb blogs, podcasts, websites, forums, videos, Facebook groups, Twitter accounts, and any other sources you have for nutrition, health, and fitness information. *Take a break.*

Use the time to get back into some other area of interest. Allow yourself to get back into a hobby or pursue a passion you've been neglecting in favor of throwing yourself 100% into keto-related media. Maybe it's art, or music, or model trains, astronomy, ancient history, or *something else* besides the exact ratios of protein, fat, and carbohydrate that are going to make the keto magic happen for you this very instant.

The nice thing about an Information Vacation is that *you won't miss a thing.*

The beauty of the internet is that every word, every link, every recording, and every controversy will be waiting for you when you come back. None of it is going anywhere. Whether you take one day off, or three days, a week, or a *month*, everything that got posted while you were gone will still be there, safe and sound.

And anyway, after you initially went low carb, when was the last time you learned anything that was *brand new* to you? Something that fundamentally changed the way you think about all this, and caused a radical change in your diet or lifestyle? That probably happens very rarely, because the truth is, it's very rare that there *is* something new. And if there ever *is* something majorly earthshattering, something that really blows the lid off *everything*, you'll end up hearing about it anyway because it'll be on the TV news, the radio news, or splashed across the front page of every major newspaper. I assure you, even if you stay away from the internet entirely, news that would immediately and radically alter what you would put on your plate that very day would somehow reach you.

I scour nutrition news almost daily for my professional writing gigs. I can assure you, *you ain't missin' nothin'.* Whatever the clickbait headlines make it *sound* like has been discovered— *groundbreaking! For the first time in history!*—if you take the time to read the full study being referenced, 9.7 times out of 10, it makes really good lining for your hamster cage. The adage "publish or perish" means there are *a lot* of studies getting published when they really should have perished. (No, just kidding; that's not what "publish or perish" means, but it *does* suggest there's a lot of utter nonsense getting published these days, and way too many websites very happy to publicize dodgy findings in a competition to get the most likes and shares.)

Bottom line: seriously, take a break. Step away from the nutrition media, social and otherwise. Find a new interest or rediscover an old one so you're not constantly inundating yourself with conflicting information about food. *There is a remedy for information overload, and it's as simple as backing off.*

Not forever; just long enough for you to recharge and come back in a calmer frame of mind.

To readers for whom none of what I've written here applies: *No problem!* If you *don't* feel overwhelmed and confused, and you *enjoy* a nonstop tsunami of nutrition and health information crashing down upon you 24/7, *great*. No stepping away needed for you. I wrote this chapter for the people who *can* benefit from a respite. The ones who write to me so paralyzed I can see tension in the *punctuation* they use. (Four exclamation points and three question marks? Yes, I understand you're frustrated. One of each would have been enough.) *You* might not be one of these folks, but they're out there. And they need to know it's okay to walk away for a while.

To Close

I hope this book has helped you find answers to why your fat loss has been slow or stalled on a low carb or ketogenic diet. My goal was to set the record straight about how and why this way of eating works, and to bust some common myths that frequently stand in the way of people getting the fat loss results they want.

If you're still struggling and would like personalized guidance, visit my website tuitnutrition.com for details on an individual consultation.

You can also find additional information on various keto-related topics on my YouTube channel (https://www.youtube.com/channel/UCmDz-SYYhoerycynsCm7L8g/). (Click on the *videos* tab to see all the videos.)

Appendix A
The Page 4 Diet: Simple, Effective Keto Fat Loss

Do you feel totally lost and overwhelmed in the sea of conflicting info out there about keto?

Are you tired of counting macros, grams of carbs, fat, and protein, putting your food into an app or spreadsheet, and worrying obsessively about every molecule of food you eat?

Are you ready to make things *SIMPLE* and *UNCOMPLICATED?*

If so, DR. WESTMAN'S PAGE 4 DIET IS FOR YOU.

If you've spent any amount of time in the ketogenic/low carb community and you *don't* know the name Eric Westman, (check your pulse; you might be dead. Dr. Westman has been conducting clinical research on low 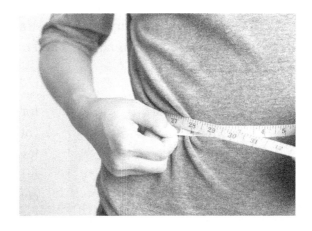 carb and ketogenic diets for 20 years. He's a co-author of the book *The New Atkins for a New You*, which he has said is the best mainstream book ever written on nutrition—not because he's a co-author, but because world-renowned, long-time keto researchers Stephen Phinney, MD, PhD, and Jeff Volek, PhD, RD, wrote the chapters on protein and fat. (His words, not mine.) Dr. Westman is also a co-author on the books *Cholesterol Clarity* and *Keto Clarity*. If you're worried about "high cholesterol" on keto, read *Cholesterol Clarity*. You won't be disappointed!

Bottom line: Dr. Westman knows his stuff. He's a past president of the Obesity Medicine Association (which has endorsed a low carb/ketogenic diet among their other strategies) and he has a 6-month waiting list at his clinic at Duke University, where he specializes exclusively in helping people use keto to lose weight and reverse type 2 diabetes, metabolic syndrome, and other related issues. **He's helped thousands of patients lose tens of thousands of pounds, and** *now the way he does it is available for you.*

Dr. Westman is famous for "page 4," which is the food list he gives his patients. In the handout he uses in his clinic, it's more like pages 4, 5 and 6, but internet shorthand for it has become "page 4." He's boiled it down to *one page – one* side of a standard 8.5 x 11" sheet of paper. It's the simplest, most straightforward, and most effective way to do keto for fat loss—and now you don't have to be his patient to get it.

> There's no guesswork, no counting, no tracking, no obsession, no fear, and no need to let your entire life revolve around what you are and are not eating. Work the plan, and the plan will work.

The Page 4 Diet calls for 20 grams *total carbs* (not net!) per day—or less. There's no nonsense, no gimmicks, and no confusion. It's a very strict form of keto, but you know what? That's why it's so effective. If it's not on page 4, *you don't eat it.* **There's no guesswork, no counting, no tracking,**

no obsession, no fear, and no need to let your entire life revolve around what you are and are not eating. Work the plan and the plan will work.

The beauty of the Page 4 Diet is that if you eat the way it says to eat, you shouldn't *need to* count anything but total carbs. You don't have to figure out macros, calories, or grams of protein and fat. You don't have to fast (but you can if you want to). You don't have to weigh, measure, or track your food. *Just stick to page 4.*

If you've been struggling with fat loss on keto for a while, this could be very helpful for you. You would likely be very surprised at what's on page 4—and maybe even more so by what's *not* on page 4. Sorry to break your hearts, but butter, heavy cream, cheese, and mayonnaise are not unlimited, and nuts aren't on the list at all. You know what you *are* told to eat as much of as you like? Meat! Meat, poultry, seafood, and eggs, so if you've been limiting protein and loading everything up with added fat instead because you've bought into the fearmongering out there about protein "turning into sugar" or "kicking you out of ketosis," it might be time for a course correction. (Visit http://www.tuitnutrition.com/2017/07/gluconeogenesis.html to read a blog post I wrote to set the record straight about protein and gluconeogenesis.)

This is a very different version of keto than you're probably used to seeing. No fat bombs, no fatty coffees, no magic ratios, no chasing ketones, and no net carbs. No shaming or judging about eating regular ol' food: doesn't have to be organic, doesn't have to be grass-fed, doesn't have to be pasture-raised or blessed by the food purity gods. It just has to be under 20 grams total carbs per day. *That's it!* You can drink diet soda, use artificial sweeteners, and eat bunless burgers or grilled chicken from fast food joints. No special membership to some pricey food delivery service required. You can get great results eating regular food from your regular supermarket, and we know you can because Dr. Westman sees this in his clinic every day.

To clarify: if whatever version of keto you're following is working for you and you're happy with the results you're getting, *keep going!* I'm sharing about the Page 4 Diet because this is a book about having difficulty losing body fat on keto, and the Page 4 Diet is an effective way to break a stall or plateau.

If this sounds intriguing to you, you can purchase the famous Page 4 Diet through my website, http://tuitnutrition.com (click on "Page 4 Keto Fat Loss.") I know ten dollars seems like a lot for *one page* of information, but I'm not kidding when I say it's the simplest and most straightforward way to do keto for fat loss. Plus, you've probably already spent *far more* on all kinds of gadgets and gizmos, books and programs, *that have failed you.* Fancy-schmancy technology, trackers, apps, and for what? To still be stymied and not understand why you're not losing weight. Now, you can get Page 4 for a relatively small investment and be on your way to keto success! That's what it is: an investment in you reaching your goals.

I'm always honest with my blog readers and video fans, and I've been honest with you throughout this book. So I want to be clear here that this is literally one page—one *side!*—of a standard sheet of paper. But it's worth every penny.

There are images and lists *claiming* to be page 4 all over Pinterest and various other places on the interwebs. *Accept no imitations!* If it didn't come from this link or from Dr. Westman himself putting it directly into your hands, I can't guarantee it's the real thing, with the version of keto he uses in his own clinic. (I would say he created it, but he credits the late and truly great Dr. Robert Atkins and the head nurse at the Atkins Center, Jackie Eberstein, for most of it. The good ol' Atkins diet is a great way to get started on keto, so if you'd rather not buy the Page 4 Diet, you can almost always find a copy of one of the Atkins books at your local library or a used book store—for free or for a handful of change. (Or get one online.) The Page 4 Diet is closely based on Atkins induction, and your results on induction will probably be just as good.

By the way: if you're wondering why page 4 is so strict—20 grams *total carbs* per day, maximum—no subtracting fiber, no subtracting sugar alcohols, no macros, no math—it's because Dr. Westman has a very broad patient base. He treats people from all walks of life and all income and education levels. Not everyone has the resources to implement a plan that requires tracking every atom of food they eat or to prick their fingers multiple times a day to measure blood sugar or ketones. Not everyone needs to live at 20 grams or fewer per day, but Dr. Westman starts everyone out that way because when carb intake is that low, you *will be* in ketosis. You *will be* burning fat. You won't *need* to measure ketones, track your food, or weigh and measure your portions—none of that.

If you stick to page 4, It. Will. Work. It is beautiful in its simplicity.

In the interest of full disclosure, I am an affiliate for Dr. Westman's Page 4 Diet, and I will receive a small percentage from each sale if you purchase it through my website.

A Note

I know...you just bought this e-book and now I'm suggesting you shell out a few more dollars for something *else?* Why didn't I just put the page 4 food list right here in my own book? Two reasons:

1. Dr. Westman created the Page 4 Diet, and it would be stealing if I were to reproduce it here.
2. So much of what we know about how the ketogenic diet works—not just for fat loss, but for type 2 diabetes, PCOS, metabolic syndrome, cardiovascular disease, irritable bowel syndrome, and more—we know because of research Dr. Westman and his colleagues have been conducting

since 1998. This was still at the height of the low-fat-whole-grains *thing*, when it took a lot of professional courage and scientific conviction to research a *high* fat diet—especially one where a lot of that fat was coming from red meat, butter, bacon, and other foods that had been demonized for decades. We owe Dr. Westman and his colleagues a debt of gratitude for sticking their necks out in those early days, and one way we can show our appreciation and support their work is to buy the Page 4 Diet. Except for the percentage that goes to affiliates, all proceeds will go toward funding more research.

Appendix B:
Dining out on a Ketogenic Diet

Provided you're careful about what you order, you can absolutely enjoy dining out while following a ketogenic diet and losing body fat. Don't be shy about customizing your order and asking for substitutions when necessary. With keto exploding in popularity and people becoming more health-conscious, not to mention the increasing prevalence of food allergies, wait staff will not be surprised or put off by special requests. They're quite familiar with the modifications you'll ask for. Servers will not look at you funny if you ask them not to bring the bread basket.

I've been eating a low carb diet for over 15 years, and I've never, *ever* been to a restaurant where there was truly nothing suitable. Saying there's nothing you can eat is a copout. Sometimes substitutions are free, sometimes they cost a few dollars more. What's staying on plan worth to you?

Here are some tips for choosing appropriate foods that will help you stick to keto at any kind of restaurant.

General Advice:

- Choose *simply prepared dishes* – grilled, baked, steamed, or roasted meats, poultry, or seafood, non-starchy vegetables, or salads. Avoid fried foods unless there's no breading or batter.

- Avoid all pasta, rice, bread, potatoes, corn, beans, soda, sugary desserts and other obvious sources of sugar and starch.

- At restaurants where free bread or rolls are provided before the food is served, request that the wait staff not bring those to the table. Ask for something else if it is the type of restaurant that is likely to have something available: sometimes olives or pickles can be served instead of starches and grains. Or better yet, just wait for your meal to be served. Let your hunger build and enjoy your entrée when it comes.

- Ask for a double portion of non-starchy vegetables in lieu of a starchy side dish. (For example, a double serving of broccoli instead of a potato, or roasted vegetables instead of pasta or rice.)

- Prepare ahead of time! Many restaurants have their menus posted online. If you're dining with other people, look in advance to see what will be suitable for you so you'll have an easier time ordering, or so you can suggest a change of location if necessary.

Tips for Specific Cuisines:

Mexican: Fajitas are a great choice—just ask the server not to bring the tortillas and ask for extra vegetables instead of rice and beans. Fajitas are just grilled meat and vegetables, and you can enjoy sour cream, cheese, guacamole, and pico de gallo as condiments. (Be sure there's no corn in the pico de gallo). At some fast food chains, you can get meat, lettuce, cheese, and vegetables in a lettuce bowl instead of a flour wrap.

Middle Eastern/Greek: Choose kebabs or other grilled meat dishes. Ask for extra vegetables or meat instead of rice or pita bread. Avoid hummus, tabbouleh, stuffed grape leaves (usually contain rice), and anything else with beans or high starch. These cuisines are famous for grilled meat specialties; take advantage of that, as well as marinated feta cheese, olives, and seared halloumi cheese. Greek salads are wonderful: lettuce, red onions, olives, feta, cucumbers, tomato—add a protein and you've got a keto meal.

Indian/Afghan/Pakistani: These are somewhat similar to the Middle Eastern cuisine discussed above. Avoid rice and bread/naan. Favor curries and dishes of grilled or roasted meat and vegetables; avoid chickpeas and potatoes.

Chinese/Japanese/Thai: Ask for your dishes to be prepared *steamed* or with *no sauce.* (Sauces typically contain sugar and corn starch. Use soy sauce or hot mustard as condiments.) Good choices for Chinese takeout are steamed chicken or shrimp with mixed vegetables. Some restaurants also offer grilled chicken or beef on skewers. Avoid rice, noodles, wontons, dumplings, deep-fried foods, and tempura (due to the breading). Sashimi is wonderful; just avoid sushi rice. For Thai restaurants, avoid noodle and rice dishes. Choose curries that contain meat or seafood and vegetables, spices, and coconut milk. Ask your server if the curries are thickened with flour or corn starch; they may be able to leave them out.

Italian: Pasta is obviously off-limits but most Italian restaurants have many other options that are perfectly fine for keto. Choose salads, steaks, chicken, pork chops, or seafood with vegetables. Avoid bread & breadsticks and ask for no croutons on your salad. Ask for extra non-starchy vegetables instead of pasta or potatoes as side dishes.

Pub/Diner/Bistro: These restaurants usually have very diverse menus and finding suitable options is easy. Just use the same logic as for anywhere else: no grains or other starchy carbohydrates, and no sweets for dessert. Fantastic choices are cobb, chef, or Caesar salads (no croutons). Bunless hamburgers or sandwiches are also fine. Always ask for non-starchy vegetables instead of fries or other potato sides. You can often substitute a simple house salad or steamed vegetables for a starchy side dish. Other good selections include any type of roasted meat, chicken, or fish, or a platter of egg or tuna salad on a bed of lettuce.

Breakfast: Stick with eggs, bacon, ham, and sausage. Avoid pancakes, waffles, potatoes, toast, bagels, muffins, fruit, juice, jam/jelly, etc. Western omelets are a great option (eggs, ham, onion, peppers), as are any type of omelets that contain eggs, meat, cheese, and/or low-starch veggies (peppers, spinach, mushrooms, onions, zucchini). Any other eggs are fine, too: poached, scrambled, over-easy, hard-boiled—however you prefer them. Avoid bottled ketchup, which contains high-fructose corn syrup. Use mustard, mayonnaise, or hot sauce as condiments.

Entrée Salads: Customize your salad as necessary: no dried cranberries, fruit, crunchy noodles, etc. Stick with lettuce, spinach, and other greens. Suitable additions are chopped hard-boiled egg, bacon, cheese, avocado, ham, turkey, chicken, steak, salmon, olives, cucumbers, sliced peppers, radishes, and other non-starchy vegetables. Use oil & vinegar or a low-carb dressing. Avoid thousand island, French, honey mustard, raspberry vinaigrette, and other high sugar dressings.

Beware of Hidden Pitfalls.

Don't be shy about asking your server for details on how foods are prepared. For example:

- Some restaurants add flour or pancake batter to their eggs to make omelets fluffier. Ask if this is the case and if so, request that they prepare your eggs without that. (One way around this is to stick with your eggs hard boiled, poached, or over-easy/sunny-side up.)

- If there's a sauce with ingredients you're not sure of, ask the server to tell you what's in it. Many sauces contain sugar, corn syrup, corn starch, and/or flour. It's best to stay with simply prepared dishes to avoid this.

- Be careful with condiments. As mentioned above, ketchup is loaded with HFCS, and many salad dressings are high in sugar and corn syrup. Your best bets for condiments (if you need them at all) are mustard (any kind except honey mustard), mayonnaise, hot sauce, melted butter, olive oil, and vinegar. (All varieties of vinegar are fine, but balsamic is a little higher in carbs.) For salad dressings, stick with ones you know are low carb, like ranch or blue cheese. (Look at labels in supermarkets to get an idea of which types are best. The carb count per 2-tablespoon serving should be 2-3 grams or less.)

Appendix C
Eating on the Go or
on the Road

Just as with dining out, you should have no trouble finding suitable options to eat if you're on the road frequently or have a hectic schedule where you're running from one task to the next and don't always have time to prepare food or sit down to a full meal. Being pressed for time or being away from your usual cooking environment does not need to be an obstacle to sticking with a low carb diet. Thanks to the expanding availability of appropriate foods just about everywhere, you'll be able to find something great no matter where you are.

Foods to grab from a quick run to a grocery store:
- Salad bar (lettuce, peppers, mushrooms, olives, chicken, ham, bacon, turkey, tuna, cheese, radishes, hard-boiled eggs, cucumbers, carrots, sunflower seeds, etc.)
- Tuna or salmon in pouches or pop-top cans
- Nuts (plain, salted or unsalted; avoid honey roasted)
- Pepperoni, salami
- Cold cuts & cheese
- Rotisserie chicken
- Pork rinds
- Deli department prepared egg salad or tuna salad

Foods to grab at a gas station or convenience store:
- Hard-boiled eggs
- String cheese, cheese sticks
- Packets of cream cheese

- Beef jerky (choose plain or original flavor – BBQ, teriyaki, and others will have more sugar)
- Nuts
- Pork rinds
- Pepperoni
- Worst case scenario: hot dogs or burgers – no bun

Foods to choose at a fast food restaurant:

- Anything that's very low in carbs!

- Bunless burgers or cheeseburgers – most fast food joints will let you order plain burger patties for a much lower price than a full burger, so if all you want is the meat for fat and protein and you don't care for the lettuce, tomato or onions, ask for plain patties.

- Bunless chicken or roast beef sandwich – choose grilled chicken if it's available, otherwise try to scrape off breading or batter.

- Salad – choose a low carb dressing and avoid salads that come with sugary ingredients like dried cranberries, crispy noodles, orange segments, etc.

- Meat and low carb vegetables over lettuce (at a Mexican or Tex-Mex chain)

In order to make sticking to a low-carb, high fat diet as easy and convenient as possible, you may want to consider keeping a supply of non-perishable foods handy in your car or desk drawer at work. Doing so will mean you're never caught in a circumstance in which you feel there is "nothing you can eat," and you opt for a high-carbohydrate item because you have no other options.

"Low carb survival pack" to keep in your car, purse, briefcase, or desk drawer:

- Pouched or canned tuna, salmon, sardines, mackerel
- Nuts, almond butter
- Beef jerky or meat-based snack bars. (Always read labels and look for brands and flavors that have little or no sugar. Some are made with dried fruit and are surprisingly high in carbs.)
- Pork rinds
- Leak-proof container of olive oil or coconut oil
- Non-perishable pepperoni, sausage or other cured meat (usually need to be refrigerated once open)

Don't forget the supplies! It does no good to have great food available if you have no way to eat it, so keep a small stash of plastic silverware, napkins, paper plates, a can opener, and plastic storage containers where you have your "emergency foods" located.

And last but not least: on the road and can't find anything keto-friendly that you're actually in the mood for? ('Cuz the truth is, you can always find something suitable. Whether or not you *want* what's available is a different story.) Consider it an opportunity to do some time-restricted eating! No harm in skipping a meal or two here and there, right? Exercise that hunger muscle a little.

References

Chapter 1

1. Feinman RD, Volek JS. Low carbohydrate diets improve atherogenic dyslipidemia even in the absence of weight loss. Nutr Metab (Lond). 2006;3:24. Published 2006 Jun 21. doi:10.1186/1743-7075-3-24.

2. Hyde P, Sapper T, Crabtree C, LaFountain R et al. Dietary carbohydrate restriction improves metabolic syndrome independent of weight loss. JCI Insight. 2019;4(12):e128308.

3. Masino SA, Rho JM. Mechanisms of Ketogenic Diet Action. In: Noebels JL, Avoli M, Rogawski MA, et al., editors. Jasper's Basic Mechanisms of the Epilepsies [Internet]. 4th edition. Bethesda (MD): National Center for Biotechnology Information (US); 2012.

4. Feinman RD, Volek JS. Carbohydrate restriction as the default treatment for type 2 diabetes and metabolic syndrome. Scand Cardiovasc J. 2008 Aug;42(4):256-63. doi: 10.1080/14017430802014838.

5. Feinman RD, Pogozelski WK, Astrup A, Bernstein RK et al. Dietary carbohydrate restriction as the first approach in diabetes management: critical review and evidence base. Nutrition. 2015 Jan;31(1):1-13. doi: 10.1016/j.nut.2014.06.011.

6. Westman EC, Tondt J, Maguire E, Yancy WS Jr. Implementing a low-carbohydrate, ketogenic diet to manage type 2 diabetes mellitus. Expert Rev Endocrinol Metab. 2018 Sep;13(5):263-272. doi: 10.1080/17446651.2018.1523713.

7. Mavropoulos JC, Yancy WS, Hepburn J, Westman EC. The effects of a low-carbohydrate, ketogenic diet on the polycystic ovary syndrome: a pilot study. Nutr Metab (Lond). 2005;2:35. Published 2005 Dec 16. doi:10.1186/1743-7075-2-35.

8. Pérez-Guisado J, Muñoz-Serrano A. The effect of the Spanish Ketogenic Mediterranean Diet on nonalcoholic fatty liver disease: a pilot study. J Med Food. 2011 Jul-Aug;14(7-8):677-80. doi: 10.1089/jmf.2011.0075.

9. Vilar-Gomez E, Athinarayanan SJ, Adams RN, et al. Post hoc analyses of surrogate markers of non-alcoholic fatty liver disease (NAFLD) and liver fibrosis in patients with type 2 diabetes in a digitally supported continuous care intervention: an open-label, non-randomised controlled study. BMJ Open. 2019;9(2):e023597. Published 2019 Feb 25. doi:10.1136/bmjopen-2018-023597.

10. Di Lorenzo C, Currà A, Sirianni G, et al. Diet transiently improves migraine in two twin sisters: possible role of ketogenesis? Funct Neurol. 2014;28(4):305–308. doi:10.11138/FNeur/2013.28.4.305.

11. Di Lorenzo C, Coppola G, Sirianni G, Di Lorenzo G et al. Migraine improvement during short lasting ketogenesis: a proof-of-concept study. Eur J Neurol. 2015 Jan;22(1):170-7. doi: 10.1111/ene.12550.

12. Barbanti P, Fofi L, Aurilia C, Egeo G, Caprio M. Ketogenic diet in migraine: rationale, findings and perspectives. Neurol Sci. 2017 May;38(Suppl 1):111-115. doi: 10.1007/s10072-017-2889-6.

13. Pointer SD, Rickstrew J, Slaughter JC, Vaezi MF, Silver HJ. Dietary carbohydrate intake, insulin resistance and gastro-oesophageal reflux disease: a pilot study in European- and African-American obese women. Aliment Pharmacol Ther. 2016;44(9):976–988. doi:10.1111/apt.13784.

14. Austin GL, Thiny MT, Westman EC, Yancy WS Jr, Shaheen NJ. A very low-carbohydrate diet improves gastroesophageal reflux and its symptoms. Dig Dis Sci. 2006 Aug;51(8):1307-12.

15. Yancy WS Jr, Provenzale D, Westman EC. Improvement of gastroesophageal reflux disease after initiation of a low-carbohydrate diet: five brief case reports. Altern Ther Health Med. 2001 Nov-Dec;7(6):120, 116-9.

16. Phillips MCL, Murtagh DKJ, Gilbertson LJ, Asztely FJS, Lynch CDP. Low-fat versus ketogenic diet in Parkinson's disease: A pilot randomized controlled trial [published correction appears in Mov Disord. 2019 Jan;34(1):157]. Mov Disord. 2018;33(8):1306–1314. doi:10.1002/mds.27390.

17. Vanitallie TB, Nonas C, Di Rocco A, Boyar K et al. Treatment of Parkinson disease with diet-induced hyperketonemia: a feasibility study. Neurology. 2005 Feb 22;64(4):728-30. doi: 10.1212/01.WNL.0000152046.11390.45.

18. Broom GM, Shaw IC, Rucklidge JJ. The ketogenic diet as a potential treatment and prevention strategy for Alzheimer's disease. Nutrition. 2019 Apr;60:118-121. doi: 10.1016/j.nut.2018.10.003.

19. Dahlgren K, Gibas KJ. Ketogenic diet, high intensity interval training (HIIT) and memory training in the treatment of mild cognitive impairment: A case study. Diabetes Metab Syndr. 2018 Sep;12(5):819-822. doi: 10.1016/j.dsx.2018.04.031.

20. Lennerz BS, Barton A, Bernstein RK, Dikeman RD et al. Management of Type 1 Diabetes With a Very Low-Carbohydrate Diet. Pediatrics. 2018 Jun;141(6). pii: e20173349. doi: 10.1542/peds.2017-3349.

Chapter 3

1. Wheless JW. History of the ketogenic diet. Epilepsia. 2008 Nov;49 Suppl 8:3-5. doi: 10.1111/j.1528-1167.2008.01821.x.

2. deCampo DM, Kossoff EH. Ketogenic dietary therapies for epilepsy and beyond. Curr Opin Clin Nutr Metab Care. 2019 Jul;22(4):264-268. doi: 10.1097/MCO.0000000000000565.

3. Masino SA, Rho JM. Mechanisms of Ketogenic Diet Action. In: Noebels JL, Avoli M, Rogawski MA, et al., editors. Jasper's Basic Mechanisms of the Epilepsies [Internet]. 4th edition. Bethesda (MD): National Center for Biotechnology Information (US); 2012.

Chapter 4

1. Ho KS, Tan CY, Mohd Daud MA, Seow-Choen F. Stopping or reducing dietary fiber intake reduces constipation and its associated symptoms. World J Gastroenterol. 2012;18(33):4593–4596. doi:10.3748/wjg.v18.i33.4593.

2. Austin GL, Dalton CB, Hu Y, et al. A very low-carbohydrate diet improves symptoms and quality of life in diarrhea-predominant irritable bowel syndrome. Clin Gastroenterol Hepatol. 2009;7(6):706–708.e1. doi:10.1016/j.cgh.2009.02.023.

3. Varjú P, Farkas N, Hegyi P, et al. Low fermentable oligosaccharides, disaccharides, monosaccharides and polyols (FODMAP) diet improves symptoms in adults suffering from irritable bowel syndrome (IBS) compared to standard IBS diet: A meta-analysis of clinical studies. PLoS One. 2017;12(8):e0182942. Published 2017 Aug 14. doi:10.1371/journal.pone.0182942.

4. Halmos EP, Power VA, Shepherd SJ, Gibson PR, Muir JG. A diet low in FODMAPs reduces symptoms of irritable bowel syndrome. Gastroenterology. 2014 Jan;146(1):67-75.e5. doi: 10.1053/j.gastro.2013.09.046.

5. Mansueto P, Seidita A, D'Alcamo A, Carroccio A. Role of FODMAPs in Patients With Irritable Bowel Syndrome. Nutr Clin Pract. 2015 Oct;30(5):665-82. doi: 10.1177/0884533615569886.

Chapter 6

1. Rowsemitt CN, Najarian T. TSH is Not the Answer: Rationale for a New Paradigm to Evaluate and Treat Hypothyroidism, Particularly Associated with Weight Loss. Thyroid Science 6(4):H1-16, 2011.

2. Rowsemitt CN. Statement on Evaluation and Treatment of Famine Response Hypothyroidism. October 2018. Personal communication.

3. Rowsemitt CN, Najarian T. Hypothyroidism, Particularly Associated with Weight Loss: Evaluation and Treatment based on Symptoms and Thyroid Hormone Levels. Thyroid Science, 6(6)CR1-7, 2011.

Chapter 7

1. Shah LM, Turner Z, Bessone SK, Winesett SP, Stanfield A, Kossoff EH. How often is antiseizure drug-free ketogenic diet therapy achieved? Epilepsy Behav. 2019 Mar 1;93:29-31. doi: 10.1016/j.yebeh.2019.01.042.

2. Felton EA, Cervenka MC. Dietary therapy is the best option for refractory nonsurgical epilepsy. Epilepsia. 2015 Sep;56(9):1325-9. doi: 10.1111/epi.13075.

3. Wheless JW. History of the ketogenic diet. Epilepsia. 2008 Nov;49 Suppl 8:3-5. doi: 10.1111/j.1528-1167.2008.01821.x.

4. Feinman RD, Volek JS. Carbohydrate restriction as the default treatment for type 2 diabetes and metabolic syndrome. Scand Cardiovasc J. 2008 Aug;42(4):256-63. doi: 10.1080/14017430802014838.

5. Feinman RD, Pogozelski WK, Astrup A, Bernstein RK et al. Dietary carbohydrate restriction as the first approach in diabetes management: critical review and evidence base. Nutrition. 2015 Jan;31(1):1-13. doi: 10.1016/j.nut.2014.06.011.

6. Westman EC, Tondt J, Maguire E, Yancy WS Jr. Implementing a low-carbohydrate, ketogenic diet to manage type 2 diabetes mellitus. Expert Rev Endocrinol Metab. 2018 Sep;13(5):263-272. doi: 10.1080/17446651.2018.1523713.

7. Westman EC, Yancy WS Jr, Mavropoulos JC, Marquart M, McDuffie JR. The effect of a low-carbohydrate, ketogenic diet versus a low-glycemic index diet on glycemic control in type 2 diabetes mellitus. Nutr Metab (Lond). 2008;5:36. Published 2008 Dec 19. doi:10.1186/1743-7075-5-36.

8. Hallberg SJ, McKenzie AL, Williams PT, et al. Effectiveness and Safety of a Novel Care Model for the Management of Type 2 Diabetes at 1 Year: An Open-Label, Non-Randomized, Controlled Study [published correction appears in Diabetes Ther. 2018 Mar 5;:]. Diabetes Ther. 2018;9(2):583–612. doi:10.1007/s13300-018-0373-9.

9. McKenzie AL, Hallberg SJ, Creighton BC, et al. A Novel Intervention Including Individualized Nutritional Recommendations Reduces Hemoglobin A1c Level, Medication Use, and Weight in Type 2 Diabetes. JMIR Diabetes. 2017;2(1):e5. Published 2017 Mar 7. doi:10.2196/diabetes.6981.

10. Mavropoulos JC, Yancy WS, Hepburn J, Westman EC. The effects of a low-carbohydrate, ketogenic diet on the polycystic ovary syndrome: a pilot study. Nutr Metab (Lond). 2005;2:35. Published 2005 Dec 16. doi:10.1186/1743-7075-2-35.

11. Palmer CM, Gilbert-Jaramillo J, Westman EC. The ketogenic diet and remission of psychotic symptoms in schizophrenia: Two case studies. Schizophr Res. 2019 Apr 6. pii: S0920-9964(19)30113-6. doi: 10.1016/j.schres.2019.03.019.

12. Kraft BD, Westman EC. Schizophrenia, gluten, and low-carbohydrate, ketogenic diets: a case report and review of the literature. Nutr Metab (Lond). 2009;6:10. Published 2009 Feb 26. doi:10.1186/1743-7075-6-10.

13. Włodarczyk A, Wiglusz MS2 Cubała WJ. Ketogenic diet for schizophrenia: Nutritional approach to antipsychotic treatment. Med Hypotheses. 2018 Sep;118:74-77. doi: 10.1016/j.mehy.2018.06.022.

14. Phelps JR, Siemers SV, El-Mallakh RS. The ketogenic diet for type II bipolar disorder. Neurocase. 2013;19(5):423-6. doi: 10.1080/13554794.2012.690421.

15. Brietzke E, Mansur RB, Subramaniapillai M, Balanzá-Martínez V et al. Ketogenic diet as a metabolic therapy for mood disorders: Evidence and developments. Neurosci Biobehav Rev. 2018 Nov;94:11-16. doi: 10.1016/j.neubiorev.2018.07.020.

16. Pérez-Guisado J, Muñoz-Serrano A. The effect of the Spanish Ketogenic Mediterranean Diet on nonalcoholic fatty liver disease: a pilot study. J Med Food. 2011 Jul-Aug;14(7-8):677-80. doi: 10.1089/jmf.2011.0075.

17. Vilar-Gomez E, Athinarayanan SJ, Adams RN, et al. Post hoc analyses of surrogate markers of non-alcoholic fatty liver disease (NAFLD) and liver fibrosis in patients with type 2 diabetes in a digitally supported continuous care intervention: an open-label, non-randomised controlled study. BMJ Open. 2019;9(2):e023597. Published 2019 Feb 25. doi:10.1136/bmjopen-2018-023597.

18. Di Lorenzo C, Currà A, Sirianni G, et al. Diet transiently improves migraine in two twin sisters: possible role of ketogenesis? Funct Neurol. 2014;28(4):305–308. doi:10.11138/FNeur/2013.28.4.305.

19. Di Lorenzo C, Coppola G, Sirianni G, Di Lorenzo G et al. Migraine improvement during short lasting ketogenesis: a proof-of-concept study. Eur J Neurol. 2015 Jan;22(1):170-7. doi: 10.1111/ene.12550.

20. Barbanti P, Fofi L, Aurilia C, Egeo G, Caprio M. Ketogenic diet in migraine: rationale, findings and perspectives. Neurol Sci. 2017 May;38(Suppl 1):111-115. doi: 10.1007/s10072-017-2889-6.

21. Pointer SD, Rickstrew J, Slaughter JC, Vaezi MF, Silver HJ. Dietary carbohydrate intake, insulin resistance and gastro-oesophageal reflux disease: a pilot study in European- and African-American obese women. Aliment Pharmacol Ther. 2016;44(9):976–988. doi:10.1111/apt.13784.

22. Austin GL, Thiny MT, Westman EC, Yancy WS Jr, Shaheen NJ. A very low-carbohydrate diet improves gastroesophageal reflux and its symptoms. Dig Dis Sci. 2006 Aug;51(8):1307-12.

23. Yancy WS Jr, Provenzale D, Westman EC. Improvement of gastroesophageal reflux disease after initiation of a low-carbohydrate diet: five brief case reports. Altern Ther Health Med. 2001 Nov-Dec;7(6):120, 116-9.

24. Obesity Algorithm®, © 2017-2018 Obesity Medicine Association. https://obesitymedicine.org/download-obesity-medicine-resources/ Accessed April 20, 2019.

Chapter 8

1. Lagraauw HM, Kuiper J, Bot I. Acute and chronic psychological stress as risk factors for cardiovascular disease: Insights gained from epidemiological, clinical and experimental studies. Brain Behav Immun. 2015 Nov;50:18-30. doi: 10.1016/j.bbi.2015.08.007.

2. Wirtz PH, von Känel R. Psychological Stress, Inflammation, and Coronary Heart Disease. Curr Cardiol Rep. 2017 Sep 20;19(11):111. doi: 10.1007/s11886-017-0919-x.

3. Gu HF, Tang CK, Yang YZ. Psychological stress, immune response, and atherosclerosis. Atherosclerosis. 2012 Jul;223(1):69-77. doi: 10.1016/j.atherosclerosis.2012.01.021.

4. van der Valk ES, Savas M, van Rossum EFC. Stress and Obesity: Are There More Susceptible Individuals? Curr Obes Rep. 2018;7(2):193–203. doi:10.1007/s13679-018-0306-y.

5. Hewagalamulage SD, Lee TK, Clarke IJ, Henry BA. Stress, cortisol, and obesity: a role for cortisol responsiveness in identifying individuals prone to obesity. Domest Anim Endocrinol. 2016 Jul;56 Suppl:S112-20. doi: 10.1016/j.domaniend.2016.03.004.

6. Gragnoli C. Depression and type 2 diabetes: cortisol pathway implication and investigational needs. J Cell Physiol. 2012 Jun;227(6):2318-22. doi: 10.1002/jcp.23012.

7. Siddiqui A, Madhu SV, Sharma SB, Desai NG. Endocrine stress responses and risk of type 2 diabetes mellitus. Stress. 2015;18(5):498-506. doi: 10.3109/10253890.2015.1067677.

8. Madhu SV, Siddiqui A, Desai NG, Sharma SB, Bansal AK. Chronic stress, sense of coherence and risk of type 2 diabetes mellitus. Diabetes Metab Syndr. 2019 Jan - Feb;13(1):18-23. doi: 10.1016/j.dsx.2018.08.004.

9. Joseph JJ, Golden SH. Cortisol dysregulation: the bidirectional link between stress, depression, and type 2 diabetes mellitus. Ann N Y Acad Sci. 2016;1391(1):20–34. doi:10.1111/nyas.13217.

10. University of California, San Francisco. Diabetes Education Online. Blood Sugar & Other Hormones. https://dtc.ucsf.edu/types-of-diabetes/type2/understanding-type-2-diabetes/how-the-body-processes-sugar/blood-sugar-other-hormones/ Accessed April 22, 2019.

11. Aronson, D. Cortisol — Its Role in Stress, Inflammation, and Indications for Diet Therapy. Today's Dietitian. Vol. 11 No. 11 P. 38.

12. Leproult R, Van Cauter E. Role of Sleep and Sleep Loss in Hormonal Release and Metabolism. Endocrine development. 2010;17:11-21.

13. Copinschi G. Metabolic and endocrine effects of sleep deprivation. Essent Psychopharmacol. 2005;6(6):341-7.

14. Van Cauter E, Knutson KL. Sleep and the epidemic of obesity in children and adults. Eur J Endocrinol. 2008;159 Suppl 1(S1):S59–S66. doi:10.1530/EJE-08-0298.

15. Knutson KL, Spiegel K, Penev P, Van Cauter E. The Metabolic Consequences of Sleep Deprivation. Sleep medicine reviews. 2007;11(3):163-178.

16. Morselli L, Leproult R, Balbo M, Spiegel K. Role of sleep duration in the regulation of glucose metabolism and appetite. Best practice & research Clinical endocrinology & metabolism. 2010;24(5):687-702.

17. Matthews KA, Dahl RE, Owens JF, Lee L, Hall M. Sleep Duration and Insulin Resistance in Healthy Black and White Adolescents. Sleep. 2012;35(10):1353-1358.

18. Javaheri S, Storfer-Isser A, Rosen CL, Redline S. The Association of Short and Long Sleep Durations with Insulin Sensitivity In Adolescents. The Journal of pediatrics. 2011;158(4):617-623.

19. Nedeltcheva AV, Scheer FAJL. Metabolic effects of sleep disruption, links to obesity and diabetes. Current opinion in endocrinology, diabetes, and obesity. 2014;21(4):293-298.

20. Reutrakul S, Van Cauter E. Interactions between sleep, circadian function, and glucose metabolism: implications for risk and severity of diabetes. Ann N Y Acad Sci. 2014 Apr;1311:151-73.

21. Reutrakul S, Mokhlesi B. Obstructive Sleep Apnea and Diabetes: A State of the Art Review. Chest. 2017;152(5):1070–1086. doi:10.1016/j.chest.2017.05.009.

22. Tasali E, Mokhlesi B, Van Cauter E. Obstructive sleep apnea and type 2 diabetes: interacting epidemics. Chest. 2008 Feb;133(2):496-506.

23. Morgenstern M, Wang J, Beatty N, et al. Obstructive sleep apnea: an unexpected cause of insulin resistance and diabetes. Endocrinol Metab Clin North Am. 2014 Mar;43(1):187-204.

24. Muraki I, Wada H, Tanigawa T. Sleep apnea and type 2 diabetes. J Diabetes Investig. 2018;9(5):991–997. doi:10.1111/jdi.12823.

25. Clarenbach CF, West SD, Kohler M. Is obstructive sleep apnea a risk factor for diabetes? Discov Med. 2011 Jul;12(62):17-24.

Chapter 9

1. Cronise RJ, Sinclair DA, Bremer AA. Oxidative Priority, Meal Frequency, and the Energy Economy of Food and Activity: Implications for Longevity, Obesity, and Cardiometabolic Disease. Metab Syndr Relat Disord. 2017;15(1):6–17. doi:10.1089/met.2016.0108.

Chapter 10

1. Gibas MK1, Gibas KJ. Induced and controlled dietary ketosis as a regulator of obesity and metabolic syndrome pathologies. Diabetes Metab Syndr. 2017 Nov;11 Suppl 1:S385-S390. doi: 10.1016/j.dsx.2017.03.022.

2. El Bacha, T., Luz, M. & Da Poian, A. (2010) Dynamic Adaptation of Nutrient Utilization in Humans. Nature Education 3(9):8.

3. Volek JS, Freidenreich DJ, Saenz C, Kunces LJ et al. Metabolic characteristics of keto-adapted ultra-endurance runners. Metabolism. 2016 Mar;65(3):100-10. doi: 10.1016/j.metabol.2015.10.028.

4. Kolata G. After 'The Biggest Loser,' Their Bodies Fought to Regain Weight. The New York Times. May 2, 2016.

5. Doyle K. 6 Years after The Biggest Loser, Metabolism Is Slower and Weight Is Back Up. Scientific American.

6. Blumenthal JA, Smith PJ, Hoffman BM. Is Exercise a Viable Treatment for Depression? ACSMs Health Fit J. 2012;16(4):14–21. doi:10.1249/01.FIT.0000416000.09526.eb.

7. Small G. Can Exercise Cure Depression? Psychology Today. Sept 25, 2010.

Chapter 11

1. Hutchison AT, Regmi P, Manoogian ENC, Fleischer JG et al. Time-Restricted Feeding Improves Glucose Tolerance in Men at Risk for Type 2 Diabetes: A Randomized Crossover Trial. Obesity (Silver Spring). 2019 May;27(5):724-732. doi: 10.1002/oby.22449.

2. Jessen NA, Munk AS, Lundgaard I, Nedergaard M. The Glymphatic System: A Beginner's Guide. Neurochem Res. 2015;40(12):2583–2599. doi:10.1007/s11064-015-1581-6.

3. Tarasoff-Conway JM et al. Clearance systems in the brain—implications for Alzheimer disease. Nature Reviews. Neurology 11, no. (8) (2015): 457-470. DOI: 10.1038/nrneurol.2015.119.

4. Mendelsohn AR, Larrick JW. Sleep facilitates clearance of metabolites from the brain: glymphatic function in aging and neurodegenerative diseases. Rejuvenation Research 16, no. 6 (2013): 518-23. DOI: 10.1089/rej.2013.1530.

Image Credits

Page #	Source website	artist
cover	shutterstock.com/	Jenn Huis
cover	istock.com/	wildpixel
3	istock.com/	Highwaystarz photography
7	istock.com/	AudreyPopov
17	tednaiman.com	Ted Naiman
18	istock.com/	monkeybusinessimages
23	istock.com/	Ildo Frazao
31	istock.com/	JacobLund
35	Pixabay.com/	Peggy and Marco Lachmann-Anlee
45	Pixabay.com/	stevebb
51	istock.com/	pogrebkov
55	istock.com/	Kwangmoozaa
61	istock.com/	Yelena Yemchuk
65	istock.com/	whitestorm
70	istock.com/	Thitaree Sarmkasat
79	istock.com/	Nauma
86	istock.com/	ttsz
86	istock.com/	Newannyart
109	istock.com/	peopleimages
116	istock.com/	samthomas
125	Pixabay.com/	congerdesign
131	istock.com/	bhofack2
133	istock.com/	Audrey Elkin
137	istock.com/	Motortion
143	istock.com/	Rawpixel
145	istock.com/	everydayplus
159	istock.com/	SI photography
161	istock.com/	Rawpixel
165	istock.com/	champja

About the Author

Amy Berger, MS, CNS, is a U.S. Air Force veteran and Certified Nutrition Specialist who specializes in using low-carbohydrate and ketogenic nutrition to help people reclaim their vitality through eating delicious foods, and showing them that getting and staying well don't require starvation, deprivation, or living at the gym. Her motto is "Keto Without the Crazy!"™ She has a master's degree in human nutrition and blogs at www. tuitnutrition.com, where she writes

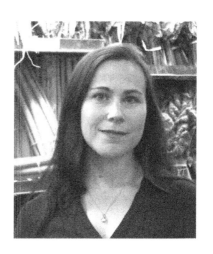

about a wide range of health and nutrition-related topics, such as insulin, metabolism, weight loss, diabetes, thyroid function, and more. She has presented internationally on these issues and is the author of *The Alzheimer's Antidote: Using a Low-Carb, High-Fat Diet to Fight Alzheimer's Disease, Memory Loss, and Cognitive Decline.*

Where to find Amy:

Website:	http://www.tuitnutrition.com/
Books:	*The Alzheimer's Antidote* (available from Amazon or request it from your local bookseller)
YouTube:	Channel name: Tuit Nutrition
Twitter:	@TuitNutrition

Visit

www.tuitnutrition.com

for more information about ketogenic nutrition and to purchase my book on Alzheimer's disease:

The Alzheimer's Antidote

AMY BERGER, MS, CNS, NTP

Foreword by David Perlmutter, MD

THE
Alzheimer's
ANTIDOTE

Using a Low-Carb, High-Fat Diet to

Fight Alzheimer's Disease, Memory Loss,

and Cognitive Decline

A Comprehensive Metabolic & Lifestyle Approach

Made in United States
Orlando, FL
28 May 2024

47286222R00108